Current Therapy and Surgery for Urogenital Tuberculosis

Ekaterina Kulchavenya

Current Therapy and Surgery for Urogenital Tuberculosis

Springer

Ekaterina Kulchavenya
Research TB Institute
Novosibirsk Medical University
Novosibirsk, Russia

ISBN 978-3-319-28288-6 ISBN 978-3-319-28290-9 (eBook)
DOI 10.1007/978-3-319-28290-9

Library of Congress Control Number: 2015959924

Printed on acid-free paper

This Springer imprint is published by SpringerNature
The registered company is Springer International Publishing AG Switzerland.

Contents

Abbreviations

AIDS	Acquired immunodeficiency syndrome
ART	Antiretroviral therapy
BCG	Bacillus Calmette–Guérin
EPTB	Extrapulmonary tuberculosis
ETTB	Extrathoracal tuberculosis
FGTB	Female genital tuberculosis
FNAC	Fine needle aspiration cytology
gUGTB	Generalized urogenital tuberculosis
HCV	Hepatitis C virus
HIV	Human immunodeficiency virus
IGRA	interferon-gamma release assay
INH	Isonicotinic acid hydrazide/isoniazid
IVU	Intravenous urography
KTB	Kidney tuberculosis
LTBI	Latent tuberculosis infection
MDR	Multidrug-resistant (TB, resistant to at least isoniazid and rifampicin)
MGM	Molecular genetic methods
MGTB	Male genital tuberculosis
Mtb	*Mycobacterium tuberculosis*
PCR	Polymerase chain reaction
PTB	Pulmonary tuberculosis
TB	Tuberculosis
TST	Tuberculin skin test
UGTB	Urogenital tuberculosis
UTI	Urogenital tract infection
UTTB	Urinary tract tuberculosis
WHO	World Health Organization

XDR Extensively drug-resistant TB (defined as resistance to at least rifampicin and isoniazid from among the first-line anti-TB drugs, in addition to resistance to any fluoroquinolone, and to at least one of three injectable second-line anti-TB drugs used in TB treatment) (capreomycin, kanamicin and amikacin)
Z-N Ziehl–Neelsen

Chapter 1
Enigmatic Tendency of Epidemiology of Extrapulmonary Tuberculosis

Abstract Extrapulmonary tuberculosis (EPTB) is an important component of tuberculosis (TB) taken as a whole, but it is often underestimated. Before we can make a reliable estimation of the epidemiology of EPTB, and particularly urogenital tuberculosis (UGTB), unification of the terminology is necessary. The term "Urogenital tuberculosis" is obviously preferable to "Genitourinary tuberculosis". Some authors understand the term "Extrapulmonary tuberculosis" as specific TB lesions of all organs, excluding bronchus, lungs, pleura and intrathoracic broncho-pulmonal lymph nodes. Others consider pleural TB as one form of EPTB – which is a reason why different authors conclude very different proportions in the spectrum of EPTB. Enigmatic tendencies were revealed also in the distribution of patients–in neighbouring regions the incidence rate may differ significantly. Many forms of EPTB are underdiagnosed: in fact, about 25 % of patients with pulmonary (PTB) and 77 % of those who died from all localizations of TB, had prostate TB – mostly having been overlooked for a lifetime. Absence of unique terms and classifications make it difficult to formulate an accurate picture of EPTB.

Keywords Epidemiology • Extrapulmonary tuberculosis • Mycobacterium tuberculosis • Prevalence • Incidence rate

1.1 Introduction

Tuberculosis (TB) remains one of the world's deadliest communicable diseases. In 2013, an estimated 9.0 million people developed TB and 1.5 million died from the disease, 360,000 of whom were HIV-positive. About 60 % of TB cases and deaths occur among men, but the burden of disease among women is also high. In 2013, an estimated 510,000 women died as a result of TB, more than one third of whom were HIV-positive. There were 80,000 deaths from TB among HIV-negative children in the same year. An estimated 1.1 million (13 %) of the 9 million people who developed TB in 2013 were HIV-positive (WHO 2014).

About one-third of the world's population has latent TB, which means people have been infected by TB bacteria but are not (yet) ill with disease and cannot transmit the disease. People infected with TB bacteria have a lifetime risk of falling

E. Kulchavenya, *Current Therapy and Surgery for Urogenital Tuberculosis*,
DOI 10.1007/978-3-319-28290-9_1

ill with TB of 10 %. However persons with compromised immune systems, such as people living with HIV, malnutrition or diabetes, or people who use tobacco, have a much higher risk of falling ill.

In 2012, about 80 % of reported TB cases occurred in 22 countries. Some countries are experiencing a major decline in cases, while cases are dropping very slowly in others. Brazil and China for example, are among the 22 countries that showed a sustained decline in TB cases over the past 20 years. In the last decade, the TB prevalence in Cambodia fell by almost 45 %. About 450,000 people developed multidrug-resistant (MDR)-TB in the world in 2012. More than half of these cases were in India, China and the Russian Federation. It is estimated that about 9.6 % of MDR-TB cases had extensively drug-resistant (XDR)-TB (WHO 2014).

Mycobacterium tuberculosis (Mtb) has, for thousands of years, existed on Earth alongside humankind: multiple traces have been found in the bones of ancient bison, who lived 17,000 years ago. For ages mankind has payed fatal tribute to tuberculosis, and even now it accounts for about 5000 human deaths daily.

TB is a multisystemic disease with myriad presentations and manifestations; it can affect any organ or tissue, excluding only hair and nails. TB (both pulmonary and extrapulmonary) leads to male and female infertility, possibly as a sexually transmitted disease (Tzvetkov and Tzvetkova 2006; Scherban and Kulchavenya 2008; Khanna and Agrawal 2011) that explains why TB is not only a medical, but also a big social problem.

1.2 Transmission of Mtb

1. Tuberculosis is mainly an airborne infectious disease, which means that the most common route of transmission of Mtb is respiratory. Infections can be spread by coughing, sneezing, laughing, singing, or just talking.
2. The second common route is alimentary transmission – usually through milk from ill cows.
3. Iatrogenic transmission, when BCG-induced TB has developed after instillation of BCG for therapy of superficial bladder cancer.
4. Direct and indirect physical contact, including sexual, are rarer ways of transmission of infection.
5. Transplacental transmission (very rare).

Independent of the route of infection, Mtb spreads through the bloodstream and lymphatic system throughout the body (so-called primary dissemination). Of course, direct contact more often leads to skin TB, an alimentary route – to intestinal TB, and prostate TB may be a cause of genital TB in a sexual partner etc. But after respiratory contamination, lungs may remain intact, kidney or lymphonodal TB may develop, and TB meningitis after alimentary contamination is possible.

1.3 Enigmas of Extrapulmonary Tuberculosis

TB as a whole consists of PTB and EPTB. While incidence, distribution and characteristics of pulmonary TB are subject to common laws, extrapulmonary TB has its own specific features.

Prevalence of TB naturally differs from region to region depending on economic and epidemic features, but if PTB in one region is about the same, EPTB is not. In any country the majority of PTB patients are young men with infiltrative PTB; this is explained by pathogenesis of the disease. But epidemiology of EPTB is an enigma of physiatria, where there are more questions than answers. Why is there such difference between prevalence of EPTB in neighboring regions? Why is the spectrum of EPTB different? What is EPTB indeed? Should we separate EPTB as a special part of TB as a whole?

The aim of our analysis was to clarify these points and try to explain them.

A Medline/PubMed research report was published with key words "*epidemiology, extrapulmonary, tuberculosis urogenital*". This research resulted in a total of six titles with only key words "*epidemiology, tuberculosis, extrapulmonary, urogenital*". The key words "*epidemiology, extrapulmonary, tuberculosis*" appeared in a total of 963 titles. Recent articles have analyzed them critically and revealed seven enigmas of EPTB.

1.3.1 First Enigma is Incomparable Epidemiologic Data on EPTB

We have no real picture of EPTB because we don't know what EPTB actually is. One of the reasons for incorrect estimation of epidemiology on EPTB is a misadjustment in terminology. Some authors consider EPTB as TB of any organ, excluding only broncho-pulmonary lesions, so pleural TB and broncho-pulmonal lymph nodes were related to the one of the form of EPTB. Others think that division of lung and its cover pleura on two separate organs is incorrect, and ascribe both organs to PTB and instead of EPTB use a term Extrathoracal Tuberculosis (ETTB), or extrarespiratory tuberculosis. WHO has considered an extrapulmonary case of TB as a patient with TB of organs other than only the lungs (e.g. pleura, lymph nodes, abdomen, genitourinary tract, skin, joints and bones, meninges). The question is – what about bronchial TB? As pleural TB is EPTB (formally it is, of course) – bronchial TB is an extrapulmonary form too? I think this position is absurd, and pulmonary TB (or more correctly – TB of breathing system, respiratory TB) should include a disease of the lungs, pleura and bronchi – and all other organs we have to attribute as extrapulmonary ones. This opinion has been totally accepted by the Russian Federation as well as in some other countries with extensive experience dealing with TB. The absence of a unique suitable definition, absence of a unanimous understanding of what really EPTB is, leads to confusing estimations of the proportion of forms of TB.

1.3.2 Second Enigma – A Different Part of EPTB Among TB as a Whole in Different Times and in Different Regions

There was very unstable prevalence of EPTB in different times and regions. In 1984 EPTB remained a major health problem in Australia, where 24.3 % of all new TB notifications were of extrapulmonary origin (Dwyer et al. 1987). In the past century in Oklahoma a greater proportion of newly diagnosed cases of EPTB occurred in nonwhites (Snider 1975). In those days EPTB was frequent in Africa and was of great severity due to delayed diagnoses and multifocal forms (Aubry et al. 1979). In the 1980s in the city of Boston, EPTB represented 4.5 % of all new cases of active TB and tended to occur in older patients (Alvarez and McCabe 1984). In Spain EPTB increased from 30.6 % of cases in 1991–1996 to 37.6 % in 2003–2008 (García-Rodríguez et al. 2011). EPTB had an increasing rate in Turkey in 2001–2007. The reason remains largely unknown (Gunal et al. 2011). In 2009 in the USA, 73.6 % were PTB and 18.7 % were EPTB (Peto et al. 2009). In developed countries, from 2 – 10 % patients with PTB have also UGTB; in developing countries such proportion increases up to 15–20 % (Figueiredo and Lucon 2008). About 20 % of patients cured of PTB, had EPTB later, mostly–UGTB (Lenk and Schroeder 2001). We have to agree that incidence is changing depending on the country and time – but not so dramatically. I'm sure the main reason is a global mistake in the definition of the EPTB and different approaches to the diagnosis and confirmation of the disease.

1.3.3 Third Enigma – Different Spectrum of EPTB in Different Regions and in Different Time

In 1984 in Australia, the commonest sites of disease were the lymph nodes, urogenital tract, pleura and bone (Dwyer et al. 1987). In Oklahoma, the majority of EPTB forms were meningitis and lymphadenitis (Snider 1975). In the 1980s in the city of Boston, sites of involvement included lymph nodes, genitourinary tract, bone and articular sites, the meninges, peritoneum, adrenal glands, pericardium, and miscellaneous sites, in this order (Alvarez and McCabe 1984). In Spain in 2003–2008 TB lymphadenitis increased up to 27 % (García-Rodríguez et al. 2011). In Nepal common sites for EPTB were lymph nodes (42.6 %) and peritoneum and/or intestines (14.8 %) (Sreeramareddy et al. 2008). The most common types of EPTB in Turkey in 2001–2007 were UGTB (27.2 %) and meningeal TB (19.4 %) (Gunal et al. 2011). But other authors from the same region reported a little different data. Among 141 EPTB patients in Istanbul for 7 years, meningeal TB accounted for 23 %, TB lymphadenitis 21 % (Sevgi et al. 2013).

In 2009 in the USA, EPTB included lymphatic (40.4 %), pleural (19.8 %), bone and/or joint (11.3 %), genitourinary (6.5 %), meningeal (5.4 %), peritoneal (4.9 %), and unclassified EPTB (11.8 %) cases (Peto et al. 2009). In France in 2012 the most frequent clinical presentations of EPTB were lymphadenitis, pleuritis and osteoarticular TB (Mazza-Stalder et al. 2012). In some countries the rate of growth of bone&joint TB reached the leading position among EPTB (Kulchavenya et al. 2013a). Location of TB on the spine remains the most common form of skeletal TB, representing 62.2 % of all osteo-articulary locations (Didilescu and Tănăsescu 2012; Wiler et al. 2010).

In Bashkortostan, female genital TB (FGTB) prevailed in 1998–2006 years, but from 2007 the bone & joint TB was a leader among EPTB (29.5 %), then–FGTB (27.4 %), then – lymphonodal TB (17.9 %). The share of UGTB was 9.5 % only (Tuktamysheva et al. 2011). We support the idea to separate urological TB and gynecological TB (female genital TB) because it allows us to better estimate the epidemiology.

Throughout the world, high TB burden countries account for about 80 % of the world's TB cases. Vietnam is one of such countries with the biggest prevalence of TB – 100 cases among 100,000 inhabitants (Do Chau Giang 2004). Among EPTB patients UGTB only was diagnosed in 77.2 %, combination of PTB and UGTB was found in 19.2 %, and UGTB and other forms of EPTB – in 3.5 % of patients (Nguyen Phuc Cam et al. 2009).

Navarro-Vilasaró et al. (2008) reported UGTB was the third most frequent EPTB infection, following pleural and nodal involvement in Spain in 2008. In the opinion of Abbara and Davidson (2011), UGTB is the second most common form of EPTB, with more than 90 % of cases occurring in developing countries. At the same time Goth and Joshi (2004) listed this form of EPTB as "others" due to low prevalence.

1.3.4 Fourth Enigma is a Non-stable Spectrum of EPTB During a Time Period

Within the last decade the spectrum of EPTB in Siberia has changed significantly (Kulchavenya et al. 2013b). TB of the central nervous system almost doubled from 4.9 to 8.7 %, mostly due to co-morbidity with HIV. Bone and joints TB increased by about half from 20.3 to 34.5 %, and among this group TB spondylitis with neurological disorders predominated. The proportion of UGTB decreased from 42.9 to 31.7 %. On the contrary, there was a decrease of peripheral lymph nodes TB from 16.7 % in 1999 to 11.2 % in 2011. At the end of the last century ocular TB accounted for 7.4 % and in 2008 (in 2009 listed in "others") for 4.4 % of the patients with EPTB. Accordingly, in 1999 other forms of TB accounted for 7.8 % and in 2009 for 15.8 % (in 2011–13.9 %). The increase is partly due to inclusion of patients with ocular TB in this group, and partly due to better diagnosis of TB of the skin, abdominal organs, breast etc. (Kulchavenya et al. 2013a, b).

1.3.5 Fifth Enigma is the Different Prevalence of EPTB in Neighboring Regions

Fritjofsson and Kollberg (1973) analyzed the incidence of UGTB in Sweden, and found that the incidence showed geographical variation within the country. The same situation was in Hungary, where the number of new cases in one province was as high as 10 per 100,000 inhabitants per year, while in another part of the country only 2–3 cases had been reported. Unexplainable different prevalence of UGTB in the neighbor regions was found in Siberia too (Kulchavenya and Krasnov 2012)– multiple predominance of the number of EPTB cases in one regions relatively another in 20–50 km – and there is no idea for the reason of this phenomena.

1.3.6 Sixth Enigma – What Does UGTB Mean (Misunderstanding in Definitions)

The first note of urogenital TB was made by Porter in 1894 [2]; in 1937 Wildbolz [3] suggested the term genitourinary TB*c* The term urogenital TB is more correct, because kidney TB, which is usually primary, is diagnosed more often than genital TB. Actually the term "urogenital tuberculosis" is incorrect too as it collects many forms with its own clinical features and requiring its own therapy and management. UGTB joins kidney TB, urinary tract TB, male and female genital TB – and every form has its own features. The combined term "UGTB" does not allow estimation of a real epidemic picture – is it prevalence of male genital TB or kidney TB? Also a high incidence rate of kidney TB 1–2 stages is better than a low incidence rate, except when complicated forms are revealed.

1.3.7 Seventh Enigma – Different Sex and Age Ration in UGTB

Some authors have found that UGTB affects more men than women (Figueiredo and Lucon 2008; Benchekroun et al. 1998; el Khader et al. 1997; Tanthanuch et al. 2010; Nurkić 2006); others – exactly the contrary (Mazza-Stalder et al. 2012; Snider 1975; García-Rodríguez et al. 2011; Singh et al. 2011). It seems that renal TB, alike any other kidney disease, should be found more often in female patients, because menses, gravidity, and inflammation of female genitals may hinder the urine passage. Urinary stasis carries a possibility for fixation of M.tuberculosis to urothelium, and, so, for developing renal TB.

For a long time in Siberia, female patients prevailed among urological TB patients, but in 2009 gender difference disappeared, and in 2010 the proportion male : female was 0,8 : 1,0 (Kulchavenya and Krasnov 2010). In Japan male : female score was 2:1, but among UGTB patients as a whole among KTB patients, gender difference was absent (Noguchi et al. 1986). In Vietnam sex proportion was 1:1.8 in favor of females (Nguyen Phuc Cam et al. 2009). Analysis of age-gender proportion showed that girls used to be ill more often than boys – as well as old women (Noguchi et al. 1986).

Age-gender correlation in kidney tuberculosis (KTB) was estimated by Zhukova et al. (Zhukova et al. 2013). KTB 2–3 stages were diagnosed in women 1.7–2.1 times more often than in men; in KTB 1 stage and KTB 4 stage there was insignificant predomination of male patients. Age-clinical distribution of nephrotuberculosis showed the lesser level of KTB in younger patients. Predomination of middle age patients and older ones among cavernous and policavernous KTB reflects the pathogenesis of this disease – a slow progressive course under masks of another disease (Zhukova et al. 2013).

Among the 64 patients, 38 (59.4 %) were male with a mean age of 60.3±16.1 years (Hsu et al. 2011). On the contrary, Hsieh HC et al. (2006) more often diagnosed UGTB in female patients.

Real estimation of urogenital tuberculosis is impossible now. This disease is very difficult for early diagnosis. It used to hide under the guises of another disease and for ages patients were managed as "urogenital tract infections (UTI)", "urolithiasis", "recurrent cystitis" etc. So we can estimate only incidence rate, but we don't know how many patients are unrevealed.

Estimates of incidence and spectrum of extrapulmonary tuberculosis (EPTB) in Siberia have been made on the basis of the data available in the official reporting forms.

As a whole, 747 patients were stricken by EPTB in Siberia in 2012, 30.0 % among them being patients with UGTB. UGTB was overlooked for 5.6 years on average: patients were managed with misdiagnoses of pyelonephritis (27 %), cystitis (43 %), cancer (8 %) or urolithiasis (22 %). Positive smear was in 17.2 %, positive PCR results in 24.3 % and positive culture of M.tuberculosis was in 44.3 %. Young men with UGTB were sub-fertile in 54.2 % and infertile in 25.9 %, 14 patients had family UGTB.

Estimated prevalence of EPTB in Siberia is 2.0 in 10,0000 inhabitants. The share of UGTB is 30.0 %, but there is a big reservoir of non-revealed patients. It is necessary to improve the awareness of this disease both between doctor and the population. At a glance we have a small number of UGTB patients. But if UTI is a problem of one patient, UGTB, as any other TB, it has a social importance, as it is a contagious disease, ii. sexually transmitted disease, iii. leads to infertility.

1.4 Rare Cases of Extrapulmonary Tuberculosis

Some EPTB forms may be very rare and so very difficult for diagnosis cases. The search in Medline/PubMed papers with key words "urogenital tuberculosis", "rare", "unusual" resulted in 235 issues on "urogenital tuberculosis rare" and 16 issues–on "urogenital tuberculosis unusual". Very rare cases of TB as duodenal tuberculosis, TB of the pharyngeal tonsil in a child, primary TB of nasopharynx (adenoid), TB appendicitis presented with caecal perforation, pancreatic TB presenting with pancreatic cystic tumor, gastric TB, pericarditis due to multidrug resistant Mtb, TB liver abscess, TB of the spleen, TB of the breast in a man, TB of the thyroid gland, and even subcutaneous granuloma of the cheek were described (Dahiya et al. 2013; Ariel' et al. 2012; Patil et al. 2013; Elamurugan et al. 2012; Rabbani et al. 2011; Moujahid et al. 2011; Kalaç et al. 2010). Although many unusual cases of extrapulmonary TB were a part of miliary TB – primary extrapulmonary TB is possible too.

Stojanović et al. (2013) described a case of primary nasal TB. The diagnosis was established on the basis of the results of nasal mucosa biopsy. Sanehi et al. (2008) revealed TB of frontal and maxillary sinus in a 68 years old male, who presented with a swelling above his left medial canthus, with no other eye or nasal complaints. Diagnosis was established on biopsy and subsequent Ziehl-Nielsen staining of nasal swabs and tuberculin skin test.

Dahiya D et al. (2013) reported a case of duodenal TB, confirmed by biopsy. A total of five patients with gastroduodenal tuberculosis were revealed in India. As exotic site of EPTB chronic ulceration of the tongue and laryngitis was described – but actually it was a first clinical sign of asymptomatic pulmonary tuberculosis (Sah et al. 1999).

The rarest case of TB of the renal artery causing a renovascular arterial hypertension was described by Bouziane et al. (2009). In southern Taiwan among a total of 766 TB patients, 102 (13.3 %) EPTB was diagnosed, and 19.6 % of EPTB patients also had PTB. The most frequently involved EPTB site was the bone and joints (24.5 %) (Lin et al. 2009). Bouchikhi et al. (2013) have found a rare case of UGTB in a man revealed by urethral narrowing and multiple urethro-scrotal fistulas.

We have described the case of iatrogenic bladder TB as a complication of BCG-therapy for bladder cancer with an outcome in shrinking bladder (Kulchavenya et al. 2013a, b). Also we have presented the case of TB of placenta in young woman, suffering from genital TB, which was overlooked before delivery (Kulchavenya and Dubrovina 2014).

We also observed an extremely rear case of extrapulmonary tuberculosis which developed after blood transmission through a mosquito bite. A young healthy woman of 32 years was bitten by a mosquito in her bare leg. She killed the mosquito, felt severe itching and scratched the place of the bite very for some time. In 3 weeks an ulcer had appeared in this area. As this woman had no history of TB, had no contact with TB, nobody could suppose TB etiology of this ulcer. A non-steroid anti-inflammatory drug and an anti-allergic drug, as well as corticoid cream, were prescribed. But the therapy had no positive result, and in a week the local lympangoitis and lymphadenitis appeared. A biopsy was performed and TB inflammation was found by patho-histology (Fig. 1.1) as well as Mtb in tissue colored by Ziehl–Neelsen was revealed.

The patient was carefully examined, but no alternative TB localization was found. The patient was treated with isoniazid, rifampicin, pyrazinamid and streptomycin for 2 months, followed by 4 months course with isoniazid and rifampicin with only good efficiency, the outcome of the disease is presented in Fig. 1.2. Follow-up is 6 years – the patient remains well.

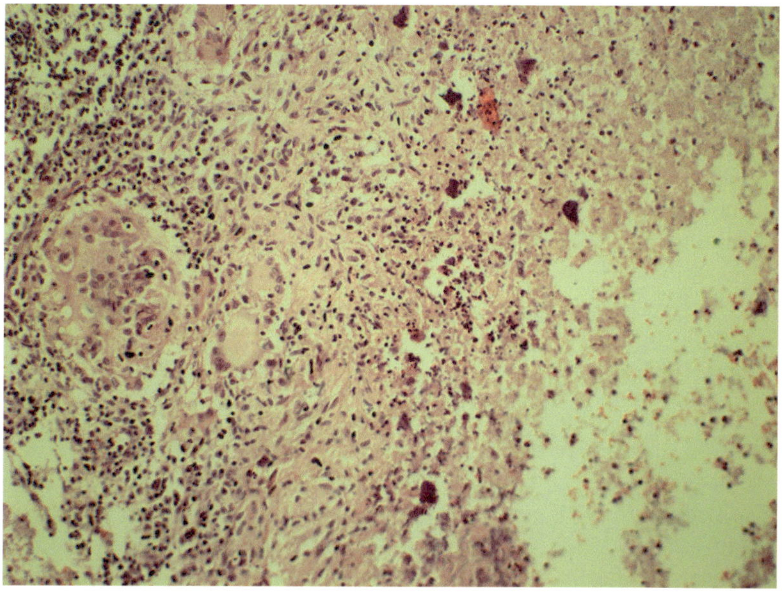

Fig. 1.1 Focus of caseous necrosis with central breakdown (*right*) in soft tissue. Epithelioid and some giant multinucleated cells around the necrosis. Note small basophilic deposits. X200. Hematoxylin and eosin

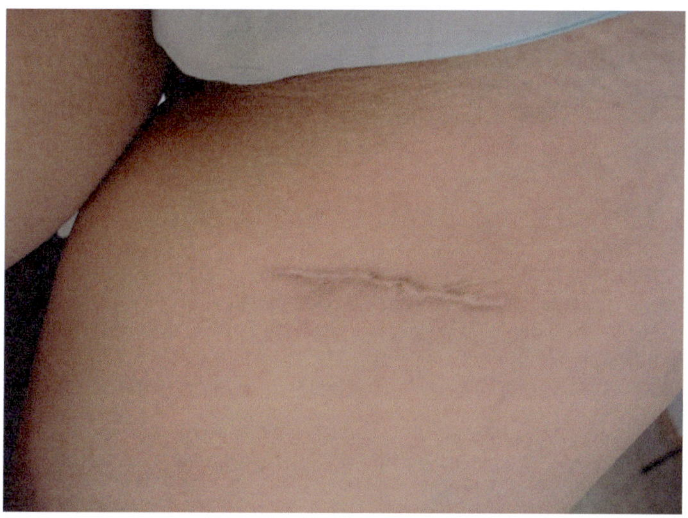

Fig. 1.2 The outcome of the disease: delicate scin scar

This patient lived in Siberia, where there is a severe epidemic situation on TB. Probably she was infected by Mtb and thus she had a latent TB, but the disease was not diagnosed. We can suppose the scenario: the stress and tissue lesion by mosquito bite provoked an activation of a dormant Mtb and active TB of skin and subcutaneous fat has developed. But we cannot exclude the exact transmission through a mosquito bite. We also can accept the hypothesis that this mosquito has bitten another patient with mycobacteriemia due to primary dissemination, and immediately thereafter this mosquito, full of infected blood, has bitten our patient, was killed and the infection has spread in the wound that led to local extrapulmonary TB.

This patient was managed correctly and a rare diagnosis was established in time by a doctor who was familiar with TB, as he worked in an epidemic region, and he had a high-suspicion index.

1.5 Conclusion

At least seven enigmas of EPTB were revealed in the literature. EPTB, despite a small member of patients, plays a significant role in both phthisiatry and urology. It is mostly because of a bigger frequency of fatal complications, a more severe decrease in quality of life, and more often association with HIV-infection, than PTB. Analyses in the literature has shown a big under-diagnosed part of EPTB patients. We have no real picture of EPTB because of defects of diagnostics, poor awareness of this disease, difficulties in identification of infection agents, absence of pathognomonic features etc. – but any attempt to estimate prevalence of EPTB is useful. We have to get a consensus in definition and classification of EPTB and, particularly in UGTB as one of the most common but an often overlooked, form of EPTB.

References

Abbara A, Davidson RN (2011) Etiology and management of genitourinary tuberculosis. Nat Rev Urol 8(12):678–688. doi:10.1038/nrurol.2011.172

Alvarez S, McCabe WR (1984) Extrapulmonary tuberculosis revisited: a review of experience at Boston City and other hospitals. Medicine (Baltimore) 63(1):25–55

Ariel' BM, Nasyrov RA, Baĭburina NA, Plechkov RE (2012) Tuberculosis of the pharyngeal tonsil in a child. Arkh Patol 74(6):35–38

Aubry P, Capdevielle P, Durand G (1979) Extrapulmonary tuberculosis in Africans. Med Trop (Mars) 39(2):156–163

Benchekroun A, Lachkar A, Soumana A, Farih MH, Belahnech Z, Marzouk M, Faik M (1998) Urogenital tuberculosis. 80 cases. Ann Urol (Paris) 32(2):89–94

Bouchikhi AA, Amiroune D, Tazi MF, Mellas S, Elammari JE, El Fassi MJ, Khallouk A, Farih MH (2013) Isolated urethral tuberculosis in a middle-aged man: a case report. J Med Case Rep 7(1):97. doi:10.1186/1752-1947-7-97

Bouziane Z, Boukhabrine K, Lahlou Z, Benzirar A, el Mahi O, Lekehal B, Mesnaoui A, Bensaid Y (2009) Tuberculosis of the renal artery: a rare cause of renovascular arterial hypertension. Ann Vasc Surg 23(6):786–789

Dahiya D, Garg M, Kaman L, Rana S, Rao C, Behera A (2013) Duodenal tuberculosis - a rare case report and review of literature. Pol Przegl Chir 85(8):464–466. doi:10.2478/pjs.2013.85.8.464

Didilescu C, Tănăsescu M (2012) Proportion and site distribution of extrarespiratory tuberculosis in 2007–2010 in Romania. Pneumologia 61(1):10–14

Do Chau Giang (2004) The current situation of Tuberculosis in the World and in Vietnam. Seminar on the National Antituberculous Program, pp 1–11

Dwyer DE, McLeod C, Collignon PJ, Sorrell TC (1987) Extrapulmonary tuberculosis-a continuing problem in Australia. Aust NZ J Med 17(5):507–511

Elamurugan TP, Sivashanker M, Kumar SS, Muthukumarassamy R, Kate V (2012) Primary tuberculous appendicitis presented with caecal perforation: a case report. Asian Pac J Trop Med 5(10):834–836. doi:10.1016/S1995-7645(12)60154-0

el Khader K, el Fassi J, Karmouni T, Tazi K, Ibnattya A, Hachimi M, Lakrissa A (1997) Urogenital tuberculosis. Apropos of 40 cases. Ann Urol (Paris) 31(6–7):339–343

Figueiredo AA, Lucon A M (2008) Urogenital tuberculosis: update and review of 8961 cases from the world literature/Figueiredo AA, Nature reviews. Urol 10(3):207–17

Fritjofsson A, Kollberg S (1973) The incidence of urogenital tuberculosis in Sweden. Int Urol Nephrol 5(3):291–296

García-Rodríguez JF, Álvarez-Díaz H, Lorenzo-García MV, Mariño-Callejo A, Fernández-Rial Á, Sesma-Sánchez P (2011) Extrapulmonary tuberculosis: epidemiology and risk factors. Enferm Infecc Microbiol Clin 29(7):502–509

Goth D, Joshi JM (2004) Clinical and laboratory observations of tuberculosis at a Mumbai (India) clinic. Postgrad Med J 80:97–100. doi:10.1136/pmj.2003.008185

Gunal S, Yang Z, Agarwal M, Koroglu M, Arıcı ZK, Durmaz R (2011) Demographic and microbial characteristics of extrapulmonary tuberculosis cases diagnosed in Malatya, Turkey, 2001–2007. BMC Public Health 11:154. doi:10.1186/1471-2458-11-154

Hsieh HC, Lu PL, Chen YH et al (2006) Genitourinary tuberculosis in a medical center in southern Taiwan: an eleven-year experience. J Microbiol Immunol Infect 39(5):408–413

Hsu HL, Lai CC, Yu MC et al (2011) Clinical and microbiological characteristics of urine culture-confirmed genitourinary tuberculosis at medical centers in Taiwan from 1995 to 2007. Eur J Clin Microbiol Infect Dis 30(3):319–326

Kalaç N, Sahin S, Gözü A, Samurkaşoğlu B, Yılmaz Aydın L, Nazlıgül Y, Tezer A (2010) Very rare presentation of extrapulmonary tuberculosis: primary gastric tuberculosis. Tuberk Toraks 58(3):293–296

Khanna A, Agrawal A (2011) Markers of genital tuberculosis in infertility. Singapore Med J 52(12):864–867

Kulchavenya E, Dubrovina S (2014) Typical and unusual cases of female genital tuberculosis. IDCases 1:92–94

Kulchavenya EV, Krasnov VA (2010) Selected Issue of Phthysiourology (monograph.). – Novosibirsk, “Nauka” (“Science”) – ISBN 978-5-02-023313-3

Kulchavenya E, Krasnov V (2012) Diseases of urinary bladder. Novosibirsk: “Nauka” (”Science”), 187 p. ISBN 978-5-02-019008-5.

Kulchavenya E, Zhukova I, Kholtobin D (2013a) Spectrum of urogenital tuberculosis. J Infect Chemother 19(5):880–883. doi:10.1007/s10156-013-0586-9

Kulchavenya E, Kholtobin D, Filimonov P (2013b) Mycobacterium tuberculosis and bovis as causes for shrinking bladder. J Case Rep Pract (JCRP) 3:57–61

Lenk S, Schroeder J (2001) Genitourinary tuberculosis. Curr Opin Urol 11(1):93–98

Lin JN, Lai CH, Chen YH, Lee SS, Tsai SS, Huang CK, Chung HC, Liang SH, Lin HH (2009) Risk factors for extra-pulmonary tuberculosis compared to pulmonary tuberculosis. Int J Tuberc Lung Dis 13(5):620–625

Mazza-Stalder J, Nicod L, Janssens JP (2012) Extrapulmonary tuberculosis. Rev Mal Respir 29(4):566–578

Moujahid M, Ziadi T, Lamsiah T, Ouzzad O, Kechna H, Moudden A (2011) Tuberculosis of the breast in a man. Sante 21(1):57–60. doi:10.1684/san.2011.0236

Navarro-Vilasaró M, Font B, Sala M, Prera A, Malet A, Mariscal D, Segura F (2008) Genitourinary mycobacteriosis: retrospective study of 45 cases in a general hospital. Enferm Infecc Microbiol Clin 26(9):540–545

Nguyen Phuc Cam Hoang, Le Van Hieu Nhan, Vu Le Chuyen (2009) Genitourinary tuberculosis: diagnosis and treatment (Abstract). Urology 74 (Suppl 4A), 30th Congress of the Société Internationale d'Urologie, Nov.:S241

Noguchi S, Shuin T, Kitajima N, Ishizuka E (1986) A clinical observation on urogenital tuberculosis. Hinyokika Kiyo 32(5):679–683

Nurkić M (2006) Frequency of microbiologicaly diagnosed urinary system tuberculosis in Tuzla canton area. Med Arh 60(6 Suppl 2):66–70

Patil C, Kharat Patil R, Deshmukh P, Biswas J, John B (2013) Primary tuberculosis of nasopharynx (adenoid) – a rare presentation. Asian Pac J Trop Med 6(3):246–248. doi:10.1016/S1995-7645(13)60033-4

Peto HM, Pratt RH, Harrington TA, LoBue PA, Armstrong LR (2009) Epidemiology of extrapulmonary tuberculosis in the United States, 1993–2006. Clin Infect Dis 49(9):1350–1357

Porter MF III (1894) Uro-genital tuberculosis in the male. Ann Surg 20(4):396–405

Rabbani K, Narjis Y, Difaa A, Louzi A, Benelkhaiat R, Finech B (2011) Tuberculous appendicitis. Saudi J Gastroenterol 17(4):287–288. doi:10.4103/1319-3767.82587

Sah SP, Raj GA, Bahadur T (1999) Chronic ulceration of the tongue and laryngitis: first clinical sign of asymptomatic pulmonary tuberculosis. J Infect 39(2):163–164

Sanehi S, Dravid C, Chaudhary N, Venkatachalam VP (2008) Tuberculosis of paranasal sinuses. Indian J Otolaryngol Head Neck Surg 60(1):85–87. doi:10.1007/s12070-008-0027-8. Epub 2008 Apr 3

Scherban M, Kulchavenya EV (2008) Prostate tuberculosis – new sexually transmitted disease. Eur J Sexology Sex Health 17(Suppl 1):163

Sevgi DY, Derin O, Alpay AS, Gündüz A, Konuklar AS, Bayraktar B, Bulut E, Uzun N, Sonmez E (2013) Extrapulmonary tuberculosis: 7year-experience of a tertiary center in Istanbul. Eur J Intern Med pii: S0953-6205(13)00913-8. doi:10.1016/j.ejim.2013.08.704

Singh DD, Vogel M, Müller-Stöver I, El Scheich T, Winzer M, Göbels S, Hüttig F, Heinrich S, Mackenzie C, Jensen B, Reuter S, Häussinger D, Richter J (2011) TB or not TB? Difficulties in the diagnosis of tuberculosis in HIV-negative immigrants to Germany. Eur J Med Res 16(9):381–384

Snider DE Jr (1975) Extrapulmonary tuberculosis in Oklahoma, 1965 to 1973. Am Rev Respir Dis 111(5):641–646

Sreeramareddy CT, Panduru KV, Verma SC, Joshi HS, Bates MN (2008) Comparison of pulmonary and extrapulmonary tuberculosis in Nepal- a hospital-based retrospective study. BMC Infect Dis 8:8. doi:10.1186/1471-2334-8-8

Stojanović J, Belić B, Mitrović S, Stanković P, Stojanović S, Erdevicki L, Zivić L, Arsenijević S (2013) Primary nasal tuberculosis: a case report. Vojnosanit Pregl 70(8):778–780

Tanthanuch M, Karnjanawanichkulm W, Pripatnanont C (2010) Tuberculosis of the urinary tract in southern Thailand. J Med Assoc Thail 93(8):916–919

Tuktamysheva LV, Azamatova MM, Yagafarova RK (2011) Epidemiology of extrapulmonary tuberculosis in Republic Bashkortostan. Tuberculez i bolezni legkih 192

Tzvetkov D, Tzvetkova P (2006) Tuberculosis of male genital system--myth or reality in 21st century. Arch Androl 52(5):375–381

WHO (2014) Fact sheet N°104, Reviewed March 2014, Available on http://www.who.int/mediacentre/factsheets/fs104/en/

Wildbolz H (1937) Ueber urogenical tuberkulose. Schweiz Med Wochenschr 67:1125

Wiler JL, Shalev R, Filippone L (2010) Case report and review: potts disease and epididymal tuberculosis presenting as back pain and scrotal mass. Am J Emerg Med 28(2):261.e3-6. doi:10.1016/j.ajem.2009.06.015

Zhukova II, Kulchavenya EV, Kholtobin DP, Brizhatyuk EV, Khomyakov VT, Osadchiy AV (2013) Tuberculosis of the urogenital system today. Urologiia 1:13–16

Chapter 2
Pathogenesis of Urogenital Tuberculosis

Abstract Tuberculosis (TB) is a contagious disease caused mainly by *Mycobacterium tuberculosis (Mtb); M. bovis* is a rather rare etiological agent of UGTB. After first contact with TB infection about 90 % of individuals remain healthy, although at least every third of them will be infected and, so, will have latent tuberculosis.

There is a genetically deterministic innate response on TB. A first meeting with Mtb provokes development of an aquired immune response on TB in an immunocompetent person; immunocompromise condition may disturb this process. Mtb survives inside macrophages by manipulating microbicidal functions such as phago-lysosome fusion, production of reactive oxygen species and nitric oxide, and by rendering macrophages non-responsive to IFN-gamma. Apoptosis prevents the release of intracellular components and the spread of mycobacterial infection by sequestering the pathogens within apoptotic bodies. Apoptosis of infected macrophages may result in self-recovery.

Thus there is an innate resistance of the human organism to Mtb – and it is a main reason why TB, a potentially lethal disease, doesn't destroy all mankind. Mtb itself stimulates acquired response on TB that improves the resistance of the human organism. Special vaccines increase this resistance too.

Tuberculosis used to be healed by forming a scar. Such scar is a benefit outcome for pulmonary TB – but in UGTB we receive "a desirable scarring in an undesirable place". Inappropriate therapy for TB ulcer of ureter may result in stricture and kidney death due to obstruction – even if this kidney is healed of TB. Redundant scarring of ductus deference may lead in obstructive infertility.

Keywords Urogenital tuberculosis • Phagocytosis • Macrophage • Pathogenesis • Mycobacterium tuberculosis • Innate human resustance

2.1 Introduction

There is a big family of *Mycobacterium* – but not all members of this family are pathogenic for humans. *Mycobacterium tuberculosis and M. bovis* are combined in ***mycobacterial complex;*** they are obligatory pathogens for human organisms. UGTB is caused by Mtb in 80–95 % of the patients, and *M. bovis* is also an

E. Kulchavenya, *Current Therapy and Surgery for Urogenital Tuberculosis*,
DOI 10.1007/978-3-319-28290-9_2

etiological agent of TB, because tuberculosis is an anthropozoonotic infection. Bacillus Calmette–Guérin (BCG), which are in fact attenuated M. bovis, are widely used for the therapy of superficial bladder cancer. In some conditions BCG-therapy may be complicated by iatrogenic BCG-induced UGTB – mainly bladder or prostate TB, but in rare cases even BCG sepsis was developed.

TB is an ancient disease that has plagued countries for centuries. The TB burden is estimated to have been most severe between 1750 and 1850. Tuberculosis is undoubtedly a fatal disease – but it is an infectious contagious disease that may be fully cured by special antibiotics. The World Health Organization estimates that one-third of the world's population is infected with Mycobacterium tuberculosis, forming a huge latent Mtb global reservoir and this renders the prospect of ever eliminating Mtb from the human race almost impossible.

About one-third of the world's population has latent TB, which means people have been infected by TB bacteria but they are not (may be yet not) ill with disease and cannot transmit the disease. People infected with Mtb have a lifetime risk of falling ill with TB of 10 %, however persons with compromised immune systems, such as people living with HIV, malnutrition or diabetes, or people who use tobacco, have a much higher risk of falling ill. As we said in Chapter I– UGTB is an enigmatic disease. And here we meet some unrequited questions again.

2.2 Unrequited Questions on TB

If every third person throughout the world is infected with Mtb – why will only10 % be ill, and the remaining 90 % will not? Why does one person after contact with Mtb get sick and die soon, and another remain healthy?

If special anti-TB drugs are created – why are only half of the patients cured? Why do 5000 people die every day due to tuberculosis, in spite of therapy? Is it possible to predict the outcome of this meeting with Mtb? Is it possible to prevent development of the disease after infection? There is no exact answer on these questions.

Probably there are two reasons for this paradox – different human vulnerability, susceptibility /resistance to tuberculosis and different virulent activity of Mtb and different sensitivity to anti-TB drugs.

2.3 Innate Human Resistance to Tuberculosis

In immunocompetent hosts, the bacterium may be controlled through innate immune mechanisms and/or by adaptive immunity. Recent studies have revealed numerous polymorphisms implicated in host susceptibility to TB. Innate resistance to Mtb was demonstrated by the well-known "**Lubeck disaster**".

2.3.1 *Lubeck Disaster*

Between 10 December 1929 and 30 April 1930, 251 infants born in the old Hanseatic town of Lubeck (Germany) received three doses of Bacillus Calmette–Guérin vaccine by the mouth during the first 10 days of life. Of these 251, 72 died of TB, most of them in 2 to 5 months and all but one before the end of the first year. Another 135 suffered from clinical TB but eventually recovered; and 44 became tuberculin-positive but remained well. The vaccine used was later found to have been contaminated with a Mtb strain being studied in the same lab (Wilson 1931). All children were equally infected by Mtb. Some of them died, some of them got sick with clinical TB, and 17.5 % remained healthy, because they had good innate resistance to TB. Although these children had no acquired immunity at all, as they all were new-born and had no time to train their immune system for Mtb, a rather big part of them won against dangerous infection owing to good innate immunity.

What kind of immunity is responsible for the outcome of the meeting with Mtb? Where were those 90 % of population, who were infected with Mtb but remained healthy, lucky due to acquired immune resistance to tuberculosis, or because they had strong innate resistance? Each stage of the host response to Mtb is under genetic control, including the initial encounter with Mtb by macrophages, epithelial cells and dendritic cells in the lung, provision of the inductive T-cell response, and killing Mtb by activated macrophages within granulomas (Yim and Selvaraj 2010). To switch on the acquired immunity to TB, meeting with a TB infection is necessary – either wild or vaccine. Yes, environmental factors, epidemic situation, co-morbidity etc. are important determinants of progression to tuberculosis; but there is a genetic component underlying susceptibility to TB, the basis of which may vary in different populations (Yim and Selvaraj 2010) – nobody can predict who will get sick with TB, and who will be resistant.

2.4 Acquired Human Resistance to Tuberculosis

Boom et al. (2003) noted, that a hallmark of Mtb infection is the ability of most (90–95 %) healthy adults to control infection through acquired immunity, in which antigen specific T cells and macrophages arrest growth of Mtb bacilli and maintain control over persistent bacilli. It is a sense of an acquired human immune resistance to tuberculosis. Individual susceptibility to TB probably plays a role in a frequency of relapses too. Shen et al. (2013) have revealed a higher rate of recurrent TB in patients after successful treatment than the incidence of new TB in general population. Authors suggested that patients with histories of TB must be considered as a group at risk of having active TB again despite successfully completed therapy.

2.4.1 The Role of Humoral Immunity

Humoral immunity plays only an auxiliary role. A humoral immune response is seen though not implicated in protection. Mtb are endowed with mechanisms through which they can evade the onslaught of host defense response: diminishing the ability of antigen presenting cells to present antigens to CD4(+) T cells; production of suppressive cytokines; escape from fused phagosomes and inducing T cell apoptosis (Boom et al. 2003; Raja 2004).

2.4.2 The Role of Polymorphonuclear Neutrophils

Polymorphonuclear neutrophils (PMN) are first in the infected organism to meet a infection aggressor. These are able to phagocytose and kill ingested Mtb, but are short-lived cells that constantly need to be removed from tissues to avoid tissue damage. Engulfment of Mtb-induced apoptotic PMN by macrophages initiates secretion of TNF-alpha from the macrophages, reflecting a pro-inflammatory response.

Moreover, Mtb-induced apoptotic PMN up-regulate heat shock proteins 60 and 72 (Hsp60, Hsp72) intracellularly and also release Hsp72 extracellularly. Both recombinant Hsp72 and released Hsp72 have enhanced the pro-inflammatory response to both Mtb-induced apoptotic PMN and Mtb. This stimulatory effect of the supernatant was abrogated by depleting the Hsp72 with immunoprecipitation (Persson et al. 2008).

In addition to direct bactericidal activities, such as phagocytosis and generation of reactive oxygen species (ROS), neutrophils can regulate the inflammatory response by undergoing apoptosis. Infection of human neutrophils with Mtb induces rapid cell death displaying the characteristic features of apoptosis such as morphologic changes, phosphatidylserine exposure, and DNA fragmentation (Perskvist et al. 2002).

Pretreatment of neutrophils with antioxidants markedly blocked Mtb-induced apoptosis but did not affect spontaneous apoptosis. The Mtb-induced apoptosis was associated with a speedy and transient increase in expression of Bax protein, a proapoptotic member of the Bcl-2 family, and a more prominent reduction in expression of the antiapoptotic protein Bcl-x(L). Phagocytosis of Mtb-induced apoptotic neutrophils markedly increases the production of proinflammatory cytokine TNF-alpha by human macrophages (Perskvist et al. 2002).

2.4.3 The Role of Macrophages

There are various aspects of macrophage-mycobacterium interactions. The role of macrophages in a host response is very important. Macrophages provide binding of Mtb to macrophages via surface receptors, phagosome-lysosome fusion, mycobacterial growth inhibition/killing through free radical based mechanisms such as reactive oxygen and nitrogen intermediates; cytokine-mediated mechanisms; recruitment of accessory immune cells for local inflammatory response and presentation of antigens to T cells for development of acquired immunity (Raja 2004).

Macrophages demonstrate tremendous phenotypic heterogeneity and functional plasticity which, depending on the site and stage of infection, facilitate the diverse outcomes. Moreover, host responses vary depending on the specific characteristics of the infecting Mtb strain (Guirado et al. 2013).

It was hypothesized that macrophages from individuals with different clinical manifestations of TB would have distinct gene expression profiles and that polymorphisms in these genes may also be associated with susceptibility to TB (Thuong et al. 2008).

A diverse T cell response allows the host to recognize a wider range of mycobacterial antigens presented by different families of antigen-presenting molecules, and thus greater ability to detect the pathogen (Boom et al., 2003).

Macrophages from subjects that are heterozygote, homozygote or compound heterozygote for these polymorphisms fail to undergo apoptosis and show partial or complete inhibition of mycobacterial killing. One of these non-functioning polymorphisms was significantly associated with increased susceptibility to TB disease, particularly extrapulmonary disease (Britton et al. 2007).

Pienaar and Lerm (2014) created the mathematical model of the initial interaction between Mtb and macrophages, which considers the interplay between bacterial killing and the pathogen's interference with macrophage function. This model revealed an oscillating balance between host and pathogen, but the balance was transient and varies in length, indicating that stochasticity in the bacterial population or host response could contribute to the diverse incubation periods observed in exposed individuals.

2.4.4 The Role of Apoptosis

The pathophysiology of Mtb infection is linked to the ability of a microorganism to grow within macrophages – it is an intracellular parasite. Apoptosis is a physiological programmed cell death process whose dysregulation plays an important role in some human infectious diseases. Apoptosis of the host macrophage is an important defense mechanism in mycobacterial infections, which prevents the spread of the infection. Unlike necrosis, apoptosis is a silent immunological event occurring without inflammation. Infection-induced target cell apoptosis may be a successful strategy to eliminate pathogens and assure host survival. Conversely, apoptosis inhibition could represent an adaptive mechanism for pathogen survival, while it may be beneficial for the host to initiate an effective immune response. Induction of early death of the infected cells may be one of the strategies of host defense against Mtb because macrophages go into apoptosis upon infection with Mtb, resulting in suppression of the intracellular replication (Danelishvili et al. 2003).

Apoptosis prevents the release of intracellular components and the spread of mycobacterial infection by sequestering the pathogens within apoptotic bodies (Fratazzi et al. 1999). Microarray analysis of infected human alveolar macrophages found serine protease inhibitor 9 (PI-9) to be the most prominently expressed of a cluster of apoptosis-associated genes induced by virulent Mtb. Inhibition of PI-9 by small inhibitory RNA decreased Mtb-induced expression of the antiapoptotic molecule Bcl-2 and resulted in a corresponding increase in production of caspase 3, a terminal effector molecule of apoptosis. Investigators concluded PI-9 induction within human mononuclear phagocytes by virulent Mtb serves to protect these primary targets of infection from elimination by apoptosis and thereby promotes intracellular survival of the organism (Toossi et al. 2012).

Danelishvili et al. (2003) has found, that both virulent (H37Rv) and attenuated (H37Ra) strains of Mtb were equally effective in inducing apoptosis macrophages; however, the attenuated strain – H37Ra resulted in significantly more apoptosis than the virulent strain H37Rv after 5 days of infection. In contrast, cytotoxicity of alveolar cells was the result of necrosis, but not apoptosis (Danelishvili et al. 2003). Although Mtb infection resulted in apoptosis of 14 % of the cells on the monolayer, cell death associated with necrosis was observed in 59 % of alveolar epithelial cells after no more than 5 days of infection. Fratazzi et al. (1999) also believed that the virulent Mtb strain H37Rv induces substantially less macrophage apoptosis than the attenuated strain H37Ra.

M. avium as well as Mtb replicate in human macrophages and induce apoptosis. Fratazzi et al. (1999) have shown that incubation of freshly added uninfected autologous macrophages with apoptotic M. avium-infected macrophages results in 90 % inhibition of bacterial growth. Apoptosis also prevents the release of intracellular components and the spread of mycobacterial infection by sequestering the pathogens within apoptotic bodies.

Weak macrophage activity and inefficient phagocytosis lead to uncontrolled replication of Mtb and death of phagocyte cells – and, so, dissemination of the infection on surrounding tissue. The apoptosis of the infected cells may result in self-recovery – it is one of the reasons for fragile balance between mycobacteria and humankind.

2.4.5 The Role of Proteins

In TB-induced response several types of proteins participate: macrophage receptors, such as the mannose receptor, Toll-like receptors (TLRs), the vitamin D nuclear receptor; phagocyte cytokines, such as tumor necrosis factor (TNF), interleukin-1β (IL-1β), IL-6, IL-10, IL-12, and IL-18; chemokines, such as IL-8, and other important innate immune molecules. Polymorphisms in these genes have been variably associated with susceptibility to TB among different populations (Azad et al. 2012; Wu et al. 2012). In most of the clinical cases of TB, the production of IL-12, IL-18 and IFN-gamma is increased, however, the group of relatively lower cytokine production did not respond well to the treatment. In addition, the plasma level of one of the chemokines, IP-10, was shown to be an indicator for the severity of the disease (Mitsuyama et al. 2003; Volpe et al. 2006).

2.4.6 The Role of Granulysin

Granulysin is an important defensive molecule expressed by human T cells and NK cells and has a cytolytic activity against microbes including Mtb and tumors. Expression of granulysin protein and mRNA in CD8 positive T cells in the patients infected with drug sensitive or MDR M. tuberculosis were lower than that in the healthy volunteers, suggesting that granulysin treatment might improve the TB disease in human (Kita et al. 2011).

2.4.7 The Role of Chemokines

Chemokines (CK) are potent leukocyte activators and chemoattractants and participate in granuloma formation, functions critical for the immune response to Mtb. It was hypothesized by Saukkonen et al. (2002) that infection of alveolar macrophages with different strains of Mtb elicits distinct profiles of CK, which could be altered by human immunodeficiency virus (HIV) infection. Macrophage inflammatory protein-1 alpha (MIP-1 alpha), and MIP-1 beta were the major beta-CK produced in response to Mtb infection. Virulent Mtb (H37Rv) induced significantly less MIP-1 alpha than did the avirulent strain (H37Ra), while MIP-1 beta production was about equal for both strains. Mtb-induced CK secretion was partly dependent on tumor necrosis factor alpha (TNF-alpha). MIP-1 beta suppressed intracellular growth of Mtb twofold to threefold. Thus, beta-CK contribute to the innate immune response to Mtb infection (Saukkonen et al. 2002).

Mtb and its protein and non-protein components are potent in induction of cytokines and chemokines from PMN and monocytes (Toossi 2000).

2.4.8 The Role of Nitric Oxide

Nitric oxide (NO), synthesized from l-arginine by NO synthases, is a small, diffusible, highly reactive molecule with dichotomous regulatory roles under physiological and pathological conditions. NO can promote apoptosis (proapoptosis) in some cells, whereas it inhibits apoptosis (antiapoptosis) in other cells. This complexity is a consequence of the rate of NO production and the interaction with biological molecules such as iron, thiols, proteins, and reactive oxygen species. Long-lasting production of NO acts as a proapoptotic modulator. However, low or physiological concentrations of NO prevent cells from apoptosis induced by trophic factor withdrawal, Fas, TNFalpha, and lipopolysaccharide (Chung et al. 2001).

2.5 Other Factors of the Immune Response

Iron acquisition is critical for Mtb growth. Access of Mtb to Fe may influence its growth in macrophages and dendritic cells (Olakanmi et al. 2013). Infection with Mtb is accompanied by an intense local inflammatory response which may be crucial to the pathogenesis of TB. Activation of some components of the innate immune response, such as recruitment of polymorphonuclear and mononuclear phagocytes and induction of pro-inflammatory cytokines, such as tumor necrosis factor alpha (TNF-alpha), by Mtb occurs early after Mtb infection, however, may persist as the organism establishes itself within granulomas (Toossi 2000).

Toll-like receptors (TLRs) play an essential role in the recognition of Mtb components by macrophages and dendritic cells, resulting in not only activation of innate immunity but also development of antigen-specific adaptive immunity (Fratazzi et al. 1999). Inerferon-gamma (IFN-gamma) also plays an important role in protection against TB. The cytokine that is produced from natural killer (NK) cells and dendritic cells at the early period of infection strongly induces not only macrophage activation but also development of antigen-specific IFN-gamma-producing CD4+T cells (Kawamura 2006).

2.6 Is Urine Bactericidal for Uropathogens (M. tuberculosis and E. coli)?

Urogenital tract infections are widespread. But most common infection agent – E. Coli – does not cause the disease to be obligatory. We would like to discover natural protective factors and supposed the hypothesis–whether urine has bactericidal activity for E. Coli, as most common infection agent for cystitis, and for M. tuberculosis (Mtb)?

We (Kulchavenya et al. 2014) investigated samples of urine in four groups: young healthy non-pregnant woman without sexual activity (sample 1), young healthy non-pregnant sexual active woman (sample 2), menopausal woman (sample 3) and young healthy man (sample 4) with automated BACTEC MGIT 960 system. We studied influence of urine on two strains of Mtb and two strains of E. Coli.

All voluntaries were healthy, their urinalyses were normal, with 1–3 leucocytes and none erythrocytes in the field of view in microscopy as well as by deep-stick. None of people had any urological complaints.

We estimated E.coli in concentrations of 3×10^8, 1.5×10^8, 1×10^8 and 0.75×10^8 microbial bodies / ml. After the exposure for 60 min and 24 h the growth of E. Coli was obtained on blood agar in all samples. Thus, the bactericidal effect of urine of healthy person all investigated groups on the E.coli not confirmed.

Also there was no bactericidal effect of urine concerning Mtb and H $_{37}$ Rv in three samples. One sample was contaminated by Enterobacter 10^2 CFU/ml – and in this sample there was no growth of Mtb both strains. We concluded that asymptomatic bacteriuria may be a reason of low microbiological diagnostic of UGTB.

2.7 How Mycobacteria Defends Itself?

When macrophage contacts with Mtb first, Mtb protects itself by disturbance of the lysosome mechanism. Dysfunction of the lysosome prevents the formation of phagolysosome, and absorbed intracellular Mtb cannot be destroyed. Even more – intracellular Mtb replicate, provoke the necrosis of the host-cell and enter into the intracellular space again. Intercellular space receives a large number of mediators and proteolytic enzymes that damage the surrounding tissue as well as lead to dissemination of the infection. This interaction between macrophage and Mtb on this stage is defined as incomplete phagocytosis. The further scenario depends on the organism's ability to activate macrophages and creates conditions for the completion of phagocytosis. Mtb survive inside macrophages by manipulating microbicidal functions such as phago-lysosome fusion, production of reactive oxygen species and nitric oxide, and by rendering macrophages non-responsive to IFN-gamma.

The slow growth and chronic nature of Mtb infection result in prolonged exposure to antigens, and hence further T cell sensitization. To survive in macrophages, Mtb has evolved mechanisms to block immune responses. These include modulation of phagosomes, neutralization of macrophage effector molecules, stimulating the secretion of inhibitory cytokines, and interfering with processing of antigens for T-cells (Boom et al. 2003). The relative importance of these blocking mechanisms likely depends on the stage of Mtb infection: primary infection, persistence, reactivation or active tuberculosis. The balance of the host-pathogen interaction in Mtb infection is determined by the interaction of T cells and infected macrophages. The outcome of this interaction results either in control of Mtb infection or active disease. Effective apoptosis is a base for self-recovery of TB.

2.8 Development of TB Infection

For a long time after contamination (up to 3 months) Mtb in the organism is unrecognized. This period is called "latent microbism" –the organism is infected already, but the immune system doesn't respond yet.

We have to remember – always there are two scenarios of the development of TB infections. Phagocytosed Mtb either are destroyed by the host cell (good scenario) or they multiply inside the endocytic compartment of mononuclear phagocytes (bad scenario). So TB is controlled by the cellular immune response. T-cell-mediated immunity amplifies macrophage capacities to kill and digest the bacilli. Specific alpha/beta T-cells produce several cytokines that attract and activate macrophages and additional lymphocytes, such as: interferon-gamma (IFN-gamma), tumor necrosis factor-alpha (TNF-alpha), interleukins 2, 6, and 12 (IL-2; IL-6 and IL-8). All these components play important roles in the immune response: IFN-gamma has the capacity to activate several antimicrobial properties of macrophages; TNF-alpha is a key cytokine involved in granuloma formation; IL-2, IL-6, IL-8 and IL-12 are candidate cytokines for the induction of Th1 cells. Furthermore, CD4+ and CD8+ T-cells display cytotoxic activity, which permits them to control mycobacterial growth through the destruction of the infected cells (Munk and Emoto 1995). The authors presented the evidence that clinical tuberculosis is associated with T-cell reactivity which controls the local concentrations of tubercle bacilli.

2.9 Pathogenesis of UGTB

Mtb induces vigorous immune responses, yet evades host immunity, persisting within phagosomes of the infected macrophages. The granuloma that forms in response to Mtb must be carefully balanced in terms of immune responses to provide sufficient immune cell activation to inhibit the growth of the bacilli, yet modulate the inflammation to prevent pathology (Flynn et al. 2011). Tuberculosis is a clinically heterogeneous disease because there are many scenarios by which balance between Mtb and immune cells can be maintained.

The primary form of the disease develops in the uninfected by Mtb organism. Secondary TB means the disease occurs in consequence of the relapse, re-infection or super-infection. Secondary TB is the pattern of disease that occurs in a previously sensitised host. It occurs after a latent period of months or years after primary infection. It may occur either by reactivation of latent Mtb or by re-infection. Reactivation occurs when dormant Mtb, persisting in tissues for months or years after primary infection, start to multiply. This may be in response to a trigger such as weakening of the immune system by HIV infection.

The wave of secondary dissemination may result in miliary TB, as well as leads to the development of local extrapulmonary forms of TB. Kidney TB may be as a local manifestation of primary miliary TB with involving all the organism in the infectious process (generalization of TB), or, more often – as secondary TB due to re-infection or super-infection.

A secondary wave of hematogenous dissemination delivers Mtb to renal vessels; Mtb penetrates the vessel's wall and are located in renal parenchyma in the periglobular area. Insufficient blood supply and disorder of urodynamics contribute to the development of kidney TB. Inducing inflow of macrophages results in specific granulomas formation – the 1st stage of kidney TB. The further development and outcome depend on virulence of Mtb and resistance of the human organism. To benefit the outcome, granuloma is substituted by fibrous tissue; in an unfavorable scenario, necrosis of the granulomas develops. When necrosis reaches the papilla– TB papillitis (kidney TB 2nd stage) is formed. If the granuloma of kidney parenchyma is located in the subcortical zone, a renal cavity surrounded by thick-layer fibrous capsule without communication with pyelocaliceal system (cavernous kidney TB 3rd stage) will be formed.

2.10 Outcomes of Kidney TB

Kidney TB 1st stage (TB of parenchyma)

Good outcome – full and fast recovery without any anatomical or functional sequels. Only kidney TB 1st stage may be cured by this scenario, as it is in a non-destructive form. All others have more or less sequels.

Negative outcome – progression of the TB infection and KTB-2 (if granuloma was in periglobular zone) or KTB-3 (if granuloma was in subcortical zone) development.

Kidney TB 2nd stage (TB papillitis)

Good outcome is development of post-TB fibrous deformation of the collecting system, forming of post-TB pyelonephritis.

Negative outcome is progress of destruction and forming a cavern.

Kidney TB 3rd stage (cavernous nephrotuberculosis)

Good outcome is transforming a cavern in the cyst (very rare), development of post-TB fibrous deformation of the collecting system, development of post-TB pyelonephritis.

Negative outcome – the progression of destruction and kidney TB 4th stage – poly-cavernous nephrotuberculosis development.

Kidney TB 4th stage (polycavernous nephrotuberculosis)

Good outcome is impossible; KTB-4 naturally resulted in kidney death.

We have to understand – late diagnosis makes full recovery of urogenital tuberculosis impossible: caverns of kidney or prostate survive forever, they cannot be fully cured by anti-TB drugs, and surgery is not always suitable. Some typical histological pictures of cavernous urogenital tuberculosis are shown in Figs. 2.1, 2.2, and 2.3.

Thick walls of cavern, disorder of microcirculation and caseous mass in cavern do not allow maintenance of enough concentration of antibiotics in the TB lesion and impede it's recovery.

There is one more very important point in the pathogenesis of UGTB. Tuberculosis normally is healed by forming a scar. Such a scar is a benefit outcome for pulmonary TB – but in UGTB we receive "a desirable scarring in an undesirable place". Inappropriate therapy for TB ulcer of ureter may result in a stricture and kidney

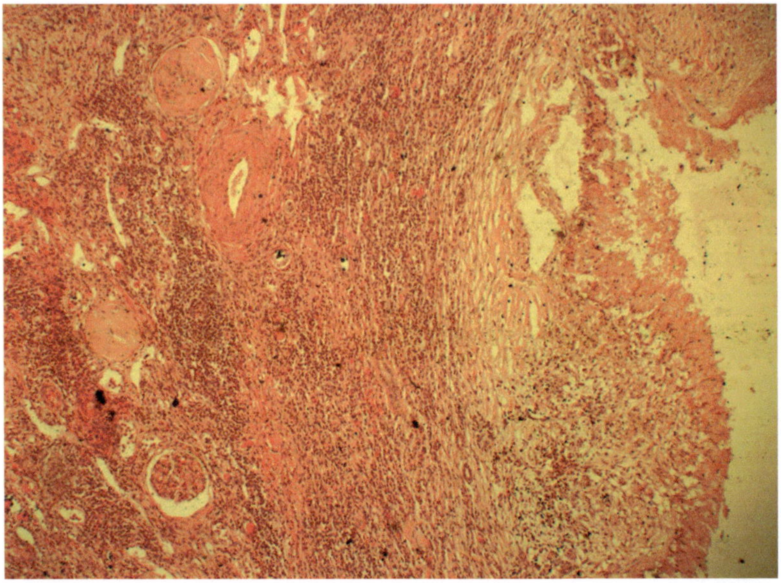

Fig. 2.1 Renal TB. The inner layer of the cavity is represented with caseous necrosis (on the *right*), deeper – epithelioid cells and immature specific granulation tissue, then mature connective tissue (forming capsule). Dense mononuclear infiltration and fibrosis of surrounded kidney tissue. Some of glomeruli are completely replaced with fibrous tissue. Tubular atrophy. ×100. Hematoxylin and eosin

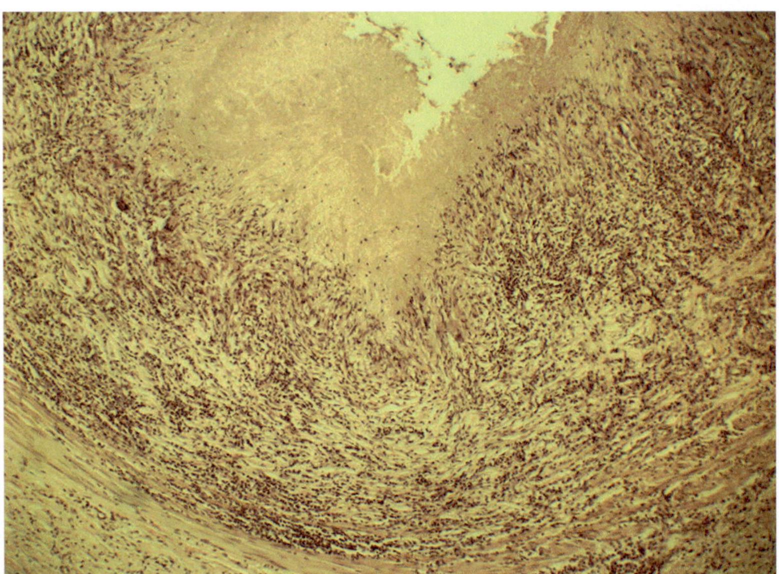

Fig. 2.2 Renal TB. Central caseation breakdown and cavity forming. ×100. van Gieson

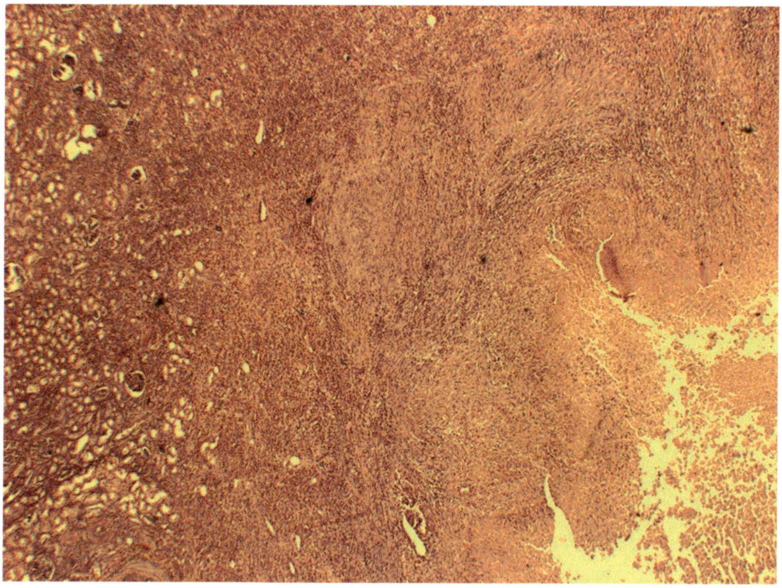

Fig. 2.3 Renal TB. Mature chronic cavity with typical three-layer wall. ×40. Hematoxylin and eosin

death due to obstruction – even if this kidney is healed of TB. Redundant scarring of ductus deference may lead in obstructive infertility. Tendency of UGTB to forming scarring is demonstrated on Fig. 2.4.

These special features of UGTB explain necessity of complex etiotropic therapy to relieve negative sequels and complications and protect an organ's function.

2.11 Vaccines Against TB Infection

To improve an acquired response on TB, special vaccines were created (Anderson and Doherty 2005). Infection of human monocytes with M. bovis BCG induced macrophage inflammatory protein (MIP)-1alpha and MIP-1beta secretion in a dose-dependent manner. The ability of M. bovis BCG to produce CC-chemokines might lead to protection in the acquired immune response of mycobacterial infection (Méndez-Samperio et al. 2003). The BCG was initially administered as a live oral vaccine. This route of administration was stopped in 1930 following the Lübeck (Germany) disaster. The intradermal route of administration was later found to be safe for mass vaccination, through studies conducted in the 1930s (Boom et al. 2003). Okada has developed a novel TB vaccine; a combination of the DNA vaccines expressing mycobacterial heat shock protein 65 (HSP65) and interleukin 12 (IL-12) delivered by the hemagglutinating virus of Japan (HVJ)-liposome or-envelope

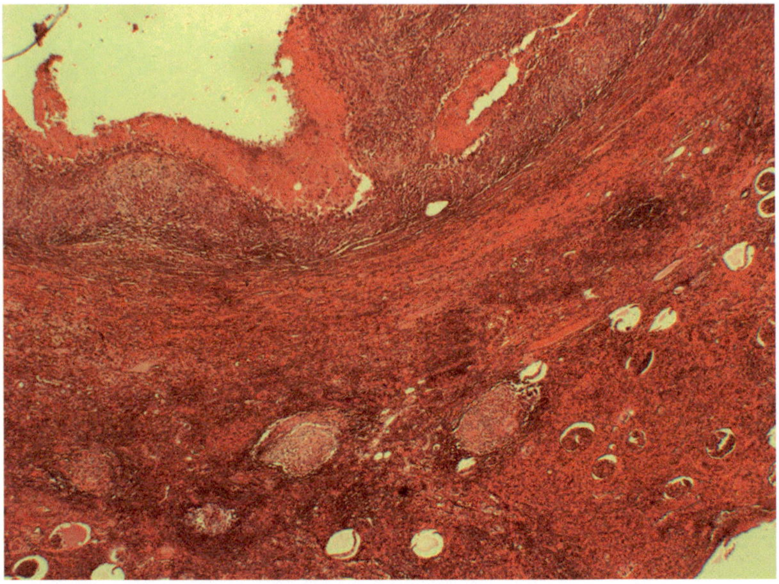

Fig. 2.4 Renal TB. Large cavity with caseous necrosis inside (*top*), surrounded by epithelioid-cell granulomata, proliferative interstitial inflammation and fibrosis. ×40. Hematoxylin and eosin

(HSP65+IL-12/HVJ). This vaccine provided remarkable protective efficacy in mouse and guinea pig models compared to the BCG vaccine, on the basis of an induction of the CD8 positive CTL activity against TB antigens and improvement of the histopathological tuberculosis lesions, respectively. The Elispot assay showed that HSP65+IL-12 DNA/ HVJ vaccine induced a greater number of IFN-gamma producing T cells than BCG in the mouse model (Okada 2008). This vaccine also provided therapeutic efficacy against multidrug resistant TB (MDR-TB) and extremely drug resistant TB (XDR-TB) in murine models (Okada 2006; Okada and Kita 2010; Okada et al. 2011).

Also recombinant virus-vectored TB vaccine was developed. A recombinant replication-deficient adenoviral (Ad) vector was engineered to express Mtb Ag85A. Single administration of this Ad vaccine via the intranasal route provided potent immune protection from pulmonary Mtb challenge. Respiratory mucosal boosting immunization with Ad vaccine was effective in enhancing T-cell activation and immune protection following parenteral DNA or BCG prime immunization (Wang et al. 2004; Xing and Lichty 2006).

Guinea pigs immunized with extracellular proteins (EP) and then challenged with aerosolized Mtb exhibit protective immunity: they were consistently protected against clinical illness, including weight loss. Actively growing Mtb release immunoprotective molecules extracellularly, that a subunit vaccine against TB is feasible; extracellular molecules of Mtb are potential candidates for a subunit vaccine (Pal and Horwitz 1992).

2.12 Conclusion

After first contact with TB infection, about 90 % of individuals may remain healthy, although some of them will be infected. The outcome of primary infection is most often a latently infected healthy human host, in whom the bacteria are held in check by the host immune response. Such individuals can develop active TB later in life with impairment in the immune system.

There is an innate resistance of the human organism to Mtb – and it is a main reason why TB, potentially lethal disease, doesn't destroy all mankind. Mtb itself stimulates acquired response on TB that improves the resistance of the human organism. Special vaccines increase this resistance too. Medical science may help to reinforce both innate and acquired response on TB, nevertheless, genetic predisposition plays important role.

References

Anderson P, Doherty TM (2005) The success and failure of BCG–implications for a novel tuberculosis vaccine. Nat Rev Microbiol 3(8):656–662

Azad AK, Sadee W, Schlesinger LS (2012) Innate immune gene polymorphisms in tuberculosis. Infect Immun 80(10):3343–3359. doi:10.1128/IAI.00443-12. Epub 2012 July 23

Boom WH, Canaday DH, Fulton SA, Gehring AJ, Rojas RE, Torres M (2003) Human immunity to M. tuberculosis: T cell subsets and antigen processing. Tuberculosis (Edinb) 83(1–3):98–106

Britton WJ, Fernando SL, Saunders BM, Sluyter R, Wiley JS (2007) The genetic control of susceptibility to Mycobacterium tuberculosis. Novartis Found Symp 281:79–89; discussion 89–92, 208–209

Chung HT, Pae HO, Choi BM, Billiar TR, Kim YM (2001) Nitric oxide as a bioregulator of apoptosis. Biochem Biophys Res Commun 282(5):1075–1079

Danelishvili L, McGarvey J, Li YJ, Bermudez LE (2003) Mycobacterium tuberculosis infection causes different levels of apoptosis and necrosis in human macrophages and alveolar epithelial cells. Cell Microbiol 5(9):649–660

Flynn JL, Chan J, Lin PL (2011) Macrophages and control of granulomatous inflammation in tuberculosis. Mucosal Immunol 4(3):271–278. doi:10.1038/mi.2011.14. Epub 2011 Mar 23

Fratazzi C, Arbeit RD, Carini C, Balcewicz-Sablinska MK, Keane J, Kornfeld H, Remold HG (1999) Macrophage apoptosis in mycobacterial infections. J Leukoc Biol 66(5):763–764

Guirado E, Schlesinger LS, Kaplan G (2013) Macrophages in tuberculosis: friend or foe. Semin Immunopathol 35(5):563–583. doi:10.1007/s00281-013-0388-2. Epub 2013 Jul 18

Kawamura I (2006) Protective immunity against Mycobacterium tuberculosis. Kekkaku 81(11):687–691

Kita Y, Okada M, Nakajima T, Kanamaru N, Hashimoto S, Nagasawa T, Kaneda Y, Yoshida S, Nishida Y, Nakatani H, Takao K, Kishigami C, Nishimatsu S, Sekine Y, Takamori Y, McMurray DN, De la Cruz EC, Tan EV, Abalos RM, Burgos JA, Saunderson P, Sakatani M (2011) Development of therapeutic and prophylactic vaccine against Tuberculosis using monkey and transgenic mice models. Hum Vaccin 7(Suppl):108–114. Epub 2011 Jan 1

Kulchavenya E, Alkhovik O, Cherednichenko A (2014) To the question of low identification of M.tuberculosis in urine. Urologia 5:53–55

Méndez-Samperio P, Vázquez A, Ayala H (2003) Infection of human monocytes with Mycobacterium bovis BCG induces production of CC-chemokines. J Infect 47(2):139–147

Mitsuyama M, Akagawa K, Kobayashi K, Sugawara I, Kawakami K, Yamamoto S, Okada Z (2003) Up-to-date understanding of tuberculosis immunity. Kekkaku 78(1):51–55
Munk ME, Emoto M (1995) Functions of T-cell subsets and cytokines in mycobacterial infections. Eur Respir J Suppl 20:668–675
Okada M (2006) Novel vaccines against M. tuberculosis. Kekkaku 81(12):745–751
Okada M (2008) The development of novel vaccines against tuberculosis. Nihon Rinsho Meneki Gakkai Kaishi 31(5):356–368
Okada M, Kita Y (2010) Anti-tuberculosis immunity by cytotoxic T cells * granulysin and the development of novel vaccines (HSP-65 DNA+IL-12 DNA). Kekkaku 85(6):531–538
Okada M, Kita Y, Nakajima T, Kanamaru N, Hashimoto S, Nagasawa T, Kaneda Y, Yoshida S, Nishida Y, Nakatani H, Takao K, Kishigami C, Nishimatsu S, Sekine Y, Inoue Y, McMurray DN, Sakatani M (2011) Novel prophylactic vaccine using a prime-boost method and hemagglutinating virus of Japan-envelope against tuberculosis. Clin Dev Immunol 2011:549281. doi:10.1155/2011/549281. Epub 2011 Mar 7
Olakanmi O, Kesavalu B, Abdalla MY, Britigan BE (2013) Iron acquisition by Mycobacterium tuberculosis residing within myeloid dendritic cells. Microb Pathog 65:21–28. doi:10.1016/j.micpath.2013.09.002. Epub 2013 Sep 22
Pal PG, Horwitz MA (1992) Immunization with extracellular proteins of Mycobacterium tuberculosis induces cell-mediated immune responses and substantial protective immunity in a guinea pig model of pulmonary tuberculosis. Infect Immun 60(11):4781–4792
Perskvist N, Long M, Stendahl O, Zheng L (2002) Mycobacterium tuberculosis promotes apoptosis in human neutrophils by activating caspase-3 and altering expression of Bax/Bcl-xL via an oxygen-dependent pathway. J Immunol 168(12):6358–6365
Persson YA, Blomgran-Julinder R, Rahman S, Zheng L, Stendahl O (2008) Mycobacterium tuberculosis-induced apoptotic neutrophils trigger a pro-inflammatory response in macrophages through release of heat shock protein 72, acting in synergy with the bacteria. Microbes Infect 10(3):233–240. doi:10.1016/j.micinf.2007.11.007. Epub 2007 Nov 29
Pienaar E, Lerm M (2014) A mathematical model of the initial interaction between Mycobacterium tuberculosis and macrophages. J Theor Biol 342:23–32. doi:10.1016/j.jtbi.2013.09.029. Epub 2013 Oct 7. Erratum in: J Theor Biol. 2014 May 21;349:172
Raja A (2004) Immunology of tuberculosis. Indian J Med Res 120(4):213–232
Saukkonen JJ, Bazydlo B, Thomas M, Strieter RM, Keane J, Kornfeld H (2002) Beta-chemokines are induced by Mycobacterium tuberculosis and inhibit its growth. Infect Immun 70(4):1684–1693
Shen X, Wu J, Jiang Y, Li J, Wang LL, Mei J, Pan QC, Gao Q (2013) Recurrent tuberculosis after successful treatment in an urban area in China. Int J Tuberc Lung Dis 17(Suppl 2,12):s98–s99
Thuong NT, Dunstan SJ, Chau TT, Thorsson V, Simmons CP, Quyen NT, Thwaites GE, Thi Ngoc Lan N, Hibberd M, Teo YY, Seielstad M, Aderem A, Farrar JJ, Hawn TR (2008) Identification of tuberculosis susceptibility genes with human macrophage gene expression profiles. PLoS Pathog 4(12):e1000229. doi:10.1371/journal.ppat.1000229. Epub 2008 Dec 5
Toossi Z (2000) The inflammatory response in Mycobacterium tuberculosis infection. Arch Immunol Ther Exp (Warsz) 48(6):513–519
Toossi Z, Wu M, Rojas R, Kalsdorf B, Aung H, Hirsch CS, Walrath J, Wolbink A, van Ham M, Silver RF (2012) Induction of serine protease inhibitor 9 by Mycobacterium tuberculosis inhibits apoptosis and promotes survival of infected macrophages. J Infect Dis 205(1):144–151. doi:10.1093/infdis/jir697. Epub 2011 Nov 16
Volpe E, Cappelli G, Grassi M, Martino A, Serafino A, Colizzi V, Sanarico N, Mariani F (2006) Gene expression profiling of human macrophages at late time of infection with Mycobacterium tuberculosis. Immunology 118(4):449–460
Wang J, Thorson L, Stokes RW, Santosuosso M, Huygen K, Zganiacz A, Hitt M, Xing Z (2004) Single mucosal, but not parenteral, immunization with recombinant adenoviral-based vaccine provides potent protection from pulmonary tuberculosis. J Immunol 173(10):6357–6365
Wilson G (1931) The Lubeck disaster. Am J Public Health Nations Health 21(3):282

Wu M, Aung H, Hirsch CS, Toossi Z (2012) Inhibition of Mycobacterium tuberculosis-induced signalling by transforming growth factor-β in human mononuclear phagocytes. Scand J Immunol 75(3):301–304. doi:10.1111/j.1365-3083.2011.02668.x

Xing Z, Lichty BD (2006) Use of recombinant virus-vectored tuberculosis vaccines for respiratory mucosal immunization. Tuberculosis (Edinb) 86(3–4):211–217. Epub 2006 Feb 28

Yim JJ, Selvaraj P (2010) Genetic susceptibility in tuberculosis. Respirology 15(2):241–256. doi:10.1111/j.1440-1843.2009.01690.x

Chapter 3
Urogenital Tuberculosis – Definition and Classification

Abstract To improve the approach to diagnose and management of urogenital tuberculosis (UGTB) we need clear and unique classification. UGTB remains an important problem, especially in developing countries, it is often overlooked disease. As any other infections, UGTB should be cured by antibacterial therapy, but because of late diagnosis it may often require surgery.

Scientific literature dedicated to this problem was critically analyzed and juxtaposed with own more than 30-years experience in TB-urology.

The conception, terms, definition were consolidated in one system; classification stage by stage as well as complication are presented. Classification of any disease includes dispersion on forms and stages and exact definition for each stage. Clinical features and symptoms significantly varied between different forms and stages of UGTB. The simple diagnostic algorithm was done.

UGTB is multivariant disease, and standard unified approach to it is impossible. Clear definition as well as unique classification is necessary for real estimation of epidemiology and optimization therapy. Join term "UGTB" has insufficient information in order to estimate therapy, surgery and prognosis – as well as to evaluate the epidemiology.

Keywords Urogenital tuberculosis • Classification • Kidney tuberculosis • Bladder tuberculosis • Male genital tuberculosis

3.1 Introduction

In 2012, the largest number of new TB cases occurred in Asia, accounting for 60 % of new cases globally (WHO 2014). UGTB is frequent form of TB, but it is a mostly overlooked disease. Despite major efforts to increase case detection, an estimated one third of new TB cases are still being missed each year, and the unavailability of a rapid, low-cost, accurate diagnostic assay that can be used at the point of care is a major hindrance (WHO 2014). There are a very few multicenter randomized studies on UGTB because of absence of unique approach to definition, diagnosis, therapy and management of this disease.

E. Kulchavenya, *Current Therapy and Surgery for Urogenital Tuberculosis*,
DOI 10.1007/978-3-319-28290-9_3

3.2 Terms and Definitions

The first note of UGTB was made by Porter in 1894; in 1937 Wildbolz suggested the term genitourinary TB. However, the term UGTB is more correct, because kidney TB (KTB), which is usually primary, is diagnosed more often than genital TB.

Urogenital tuberculosis (UGTB) – infectious inflammation of any urogenital organ – isolated or in combination (kidney and/or male or female genitals), – caused by Mtb or *M. bovis.*
Genital tuberculosis (GTB) – infectious inflammation of the female or male genitals – accordingly female genital tuberculosis (FGTB) or male genital tuberculosis (MGTB) caused by *Mtb* or *M. bovis.*
Kidney tuberculosis (KTB) – infectious inflammation of kidney parenchyma, caused by *Mtb* or *M. bovis.*
Urinary tract tuberculosis (UTTB) – infectious-allergic inflammation of calyx, pelvic and upper and lower urinary tract caused by *Mtb* or *M. bovis,* always secondary to kidney TB and should be considered as a complication of kidney TB.
Generalized urogenital tuberculosis (gUGTB) – generalized tuberculosis of the kidney and the male or female genitals, respectively.

3.3 Classifications of UGTB

UGTB includes many forms of TB with its own clinical features requiring specific therapy and management. Therefore correct clinical classification and staging are important for optimal management and therapy. UGTB can be subclassified into the following entities: kidney tuberculosis and genital tuberculosis.

3.3.1 Kidney Tuberculosis

There are four stages to be considered for **Kidney tuberculosis**:

Stage 1: TB of kidney parenchyma (non-destructive form, KTB-1).
Stage 2: TB papillitis (small-destructive form, KTB-2).
Stage 3: Cavernous kidney TB (destructive form, KTB-3).
Stage 4: Polycavernous kidney TB (widespread-destructive form, KTB-4).

Complications of kidney TB are chronic renal failure, fistula, high blood pressure.

3.3.2 Urinary Tract TB

- **TB of ureter**.
- **TB of the bladder** is divided into four stages (Kulchavenya 2010):

Stage 1 – tubercle-infiltrative;
Stage 2 – erosive-ulcerous;
Stage 3 – spastic cystitis, which in fact means overactive bladder;
Stage 4 – contracted bladder up to full obliteration.

There is one more form of bladder TB, the iatrogenic BCG-induced bladder TB, which develops as a complication of BCG therapy for bladder cancer.

- **TB of urethra.**

3.3.3 Male Genital Tuberculosis (MGTB)

- TB epididymitis (Uni- or bilateral)
- TB orchiepididymitis (Uni- or bilateral)
- TB of the prostate (infiltrative or cavernous forms)
- TB of seminal vesicles
- TB of the penis

Complications of MGTB are strictures, fistula, infertility, sexual dysfunction.
Female genital tuberculosis (FGTB) (is not included in this book).
Generalized urogenital tuberculosis (gUGTB): simultaneous lesion of the kidney and the genital organs; gUGTB is always considered as a complicated TB.

3.4 Clinical Features

Clinical features of UGTB have no specific signs, are instable and depend on many factors; this is one of the reasons for late diagnosis.

Comparison of clinical features of UGTB was conducted between 1st group, which were ill in benefit antibacterial era and 2nd group which were ill in novo days.

Current trends of UGTB have shown a change of clinical features: torpid, latent, obscure course predominates; while in the 1st group 35 % of patients had an acute onset of UGTB. Flank pain and haematuria were diagnosed significantly more often novo days. The frequency of pyuria and dysuria was the same, as well as renal colic. In the 1st group mycobacteriuria was found in 85 %, in 2nd group this symptom has decreased up to 44 %, mostly because of widespread using of antibiotics.

3.4.1 Clinical Features of Kidney TB

As whole KTB patients complain of flank pain (up to 80 %) and/or dysuria (up to 54 %). If the urinary tract is involved, then renal colic (24 %) and gross-hematuria (up to 20 %) are possible. Prostate TB manifests by perineal pain and dysuria, and

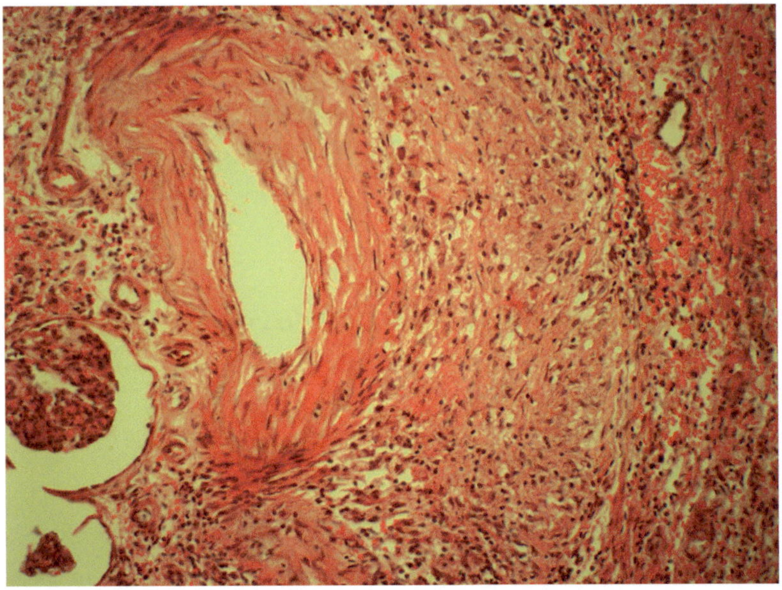

Fig. 3.1 Kidney TB. Perivascular epithelioid-cell granuloma. ×200. Hematoxylin and eosin

in half of the cases by hemospermia. TB orchiepididymitis always starts from epididymitis, isolated TB orchitis does not exist. Oedema and swelling of the scrotal organs and pain are most often the first symptoms. In 68 % there is an acute debut of the disease. Nevertheless, in 32–40 % the disease has a chronic or asymptomatic course (Figueiredo and Lucon 2008; Lenk and Schroeder 2001; Miyake and Fujisawa 2011; Carrillo-Esper et al. 2010).

- **KTB-1** has minimal lesion without destruction, full recovery is possible by anti-TB drugs. Intravenous urography (IVU) is normal. Urinalysis in children is often normal, but in adults low level leucocyturia may be found. Usually patients have no complaints and are diagnosed by chance. KTB-1 is complicated very rarely. Prognosis is good, usually outcome is full recovery. With inappropriate therapy KTB-1 may progress to destructive form. KTB-1 should be confirmed by bacteriology in any case. Usually Mtb in KTB-1 patients are sensitive to anti-Tb drugs. Mtb detection in urine is always necessary for diagnosing kidney TB stage 1, but may not always be revealed in other forms of UGTB.

If biopsy was performed – single granulomas may be found (Figs 3.1, and 3.2). Very important point – positive result of pathohistological investigation confirm diagnosis "tuberculosis", but negative result doesn't exclude it, as granulomas are localized sporadically, and zone of TB inflammation may be missed.

- **KTB-2** is subject to conservative therapy, but if KTB-2 is complicated by urinary tract TB, than reconstructive surgery is indicated. Prognosis is good; usual outcome

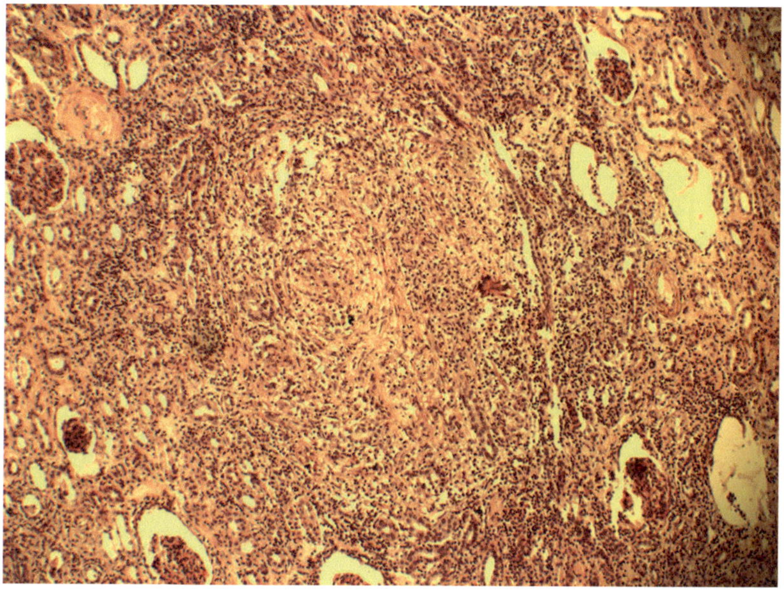

Fig. 3.2 Kidney TB. Large epithelioid-cell granuloma. ×100. Hematoxylin and eosin

is recovery with fibrous deformation and post-tuberculous pyelonephritis. With inappropriate therapy KTB-2 may progress to the next stage. Mtb is not detected in all cases and may be resistant.

Pathohistological findings – granulomas with necrosis (Fig 3.3).

- **KTB-3** has two ways of pathogenesis, from TB of parenchyma or from papillitis. The first way means development of a sub-cortical cavern without connection to the collecting system. The clinical manifestation of a sub-cortical cavern is similar to a renal carbuncle, thus the diagnosis is usually made after the operation. The second way is the destruction of the papilla until a cavern is developed. Complications develop in more than half of the patients. Full recovery by anti-TB drugs is impossible, surgery is generally indicated. The best outcome is the formation of a sterile cyst; a negative outcome is further destruction upto polycavernous TB.

Pathohistological findings–interstitial proliferative inflammation, fibrosis of the stroma and of some glomeruli, cavern with typical three-layered wall.

- **KTB-4** means several caverns in the kidney; nevertheless overall renal function may be sufficient. KTB-4 may result in fistulas due to pyonephrosis. Self-recovery is also possible, when a stricture of the ureter locks the kidney and caseation in the caverns is impregnated by calcium, the so-called auto-amputation of the kidney. KTB-4 is almost always complicated; very often the contralateral kidney is involved. Recovery with anti-TB drugs only is impossible; surgery is

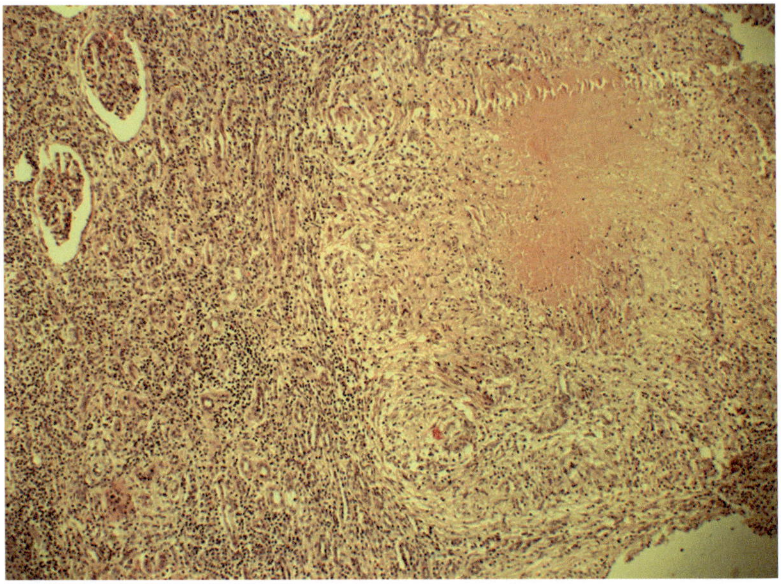

Fig. 3.3 Kidney TB. Large and small epithelioid granulomata with central caseous necrosis. ×100. van Gieson

necessary, basically nephrectomy. Diagnosis is confirmed by UVI and multislice computer tomogram, pathohistological findings may reveal caseous, fibrosis, sever inflammation (Figs 3.4, and 3.5). Removed kidney with TB 4th stage is shown on Fig 3.6.

3.4.2 Clinical Features of Urinary Tract TB

Urinary tract TB is a specific complication of KTB and so is always secondary to KTB. Urinary tract TB with any localization first appears as an oedema; the next stages are infiltration, ulceration and fibrosis.

- **TB of ureter** usually develops in the lower third, but multiple lesions are possible, too. Incorrect therapy may lead to development of a ureteral stricture which may result in loss of the kidney, even if TB is finally cured. Pathohistological findings are shown on Figs 3.7, and 3.8.
- **TB of the bladder.** The main symptom is frequency, then urgency, hematuria. The first two stages should be treated by standard anti-TB drugs; the 3-rd stage with standard anti-TB drugs and trospium chloride, and the 4-th stage is indicated for cystectomy with following enteroplasty. Bladder tuberculosis (BTB) complicates kidney TB in 45.8–84.8 % and is one of the most severe complications, and leads to the shrinking of bladder and development of terminal renal failure. To

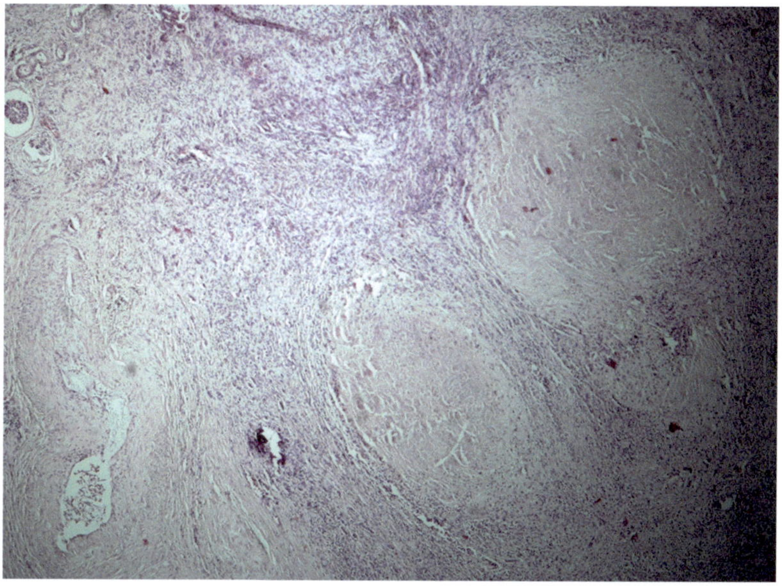

Fig. 3.4 Kidney TB 4th stage with huge caseous destruction

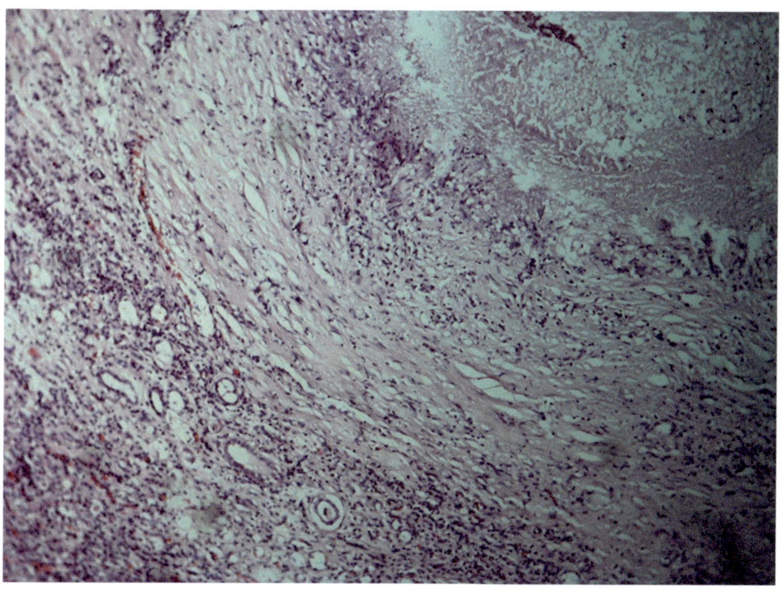

Fig. 3.5 Kidney TB 4th stage – cavern with typical three-layered wall

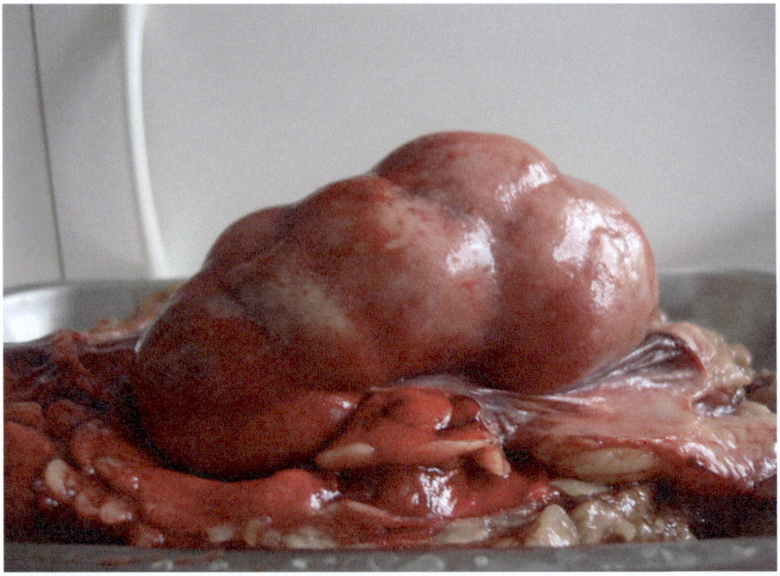

Fig.3.6 Nephrectomy due to kidney TB 4th stage – many huge caverns

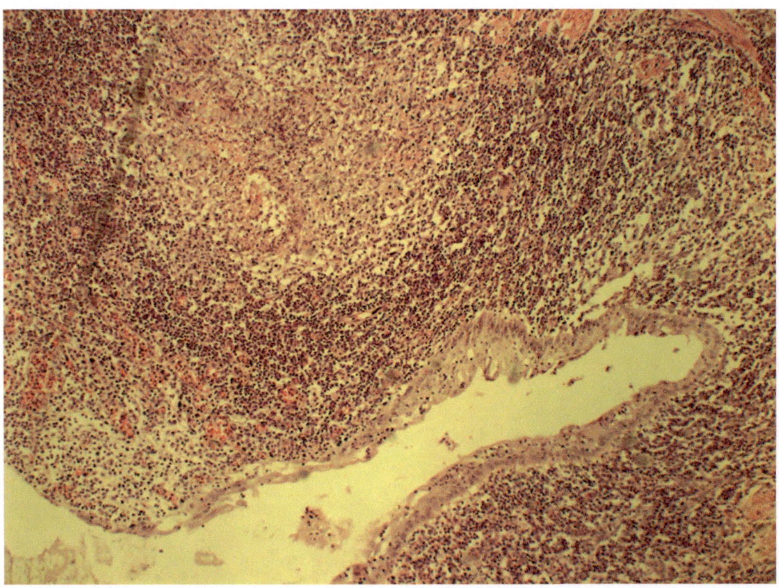

Fig. 3.7 TB of ureter. Arround the mucous membrane – epithelioid-cell granulomata, dense lymphoid infiltration. ×100. Hematoxylin and eosin

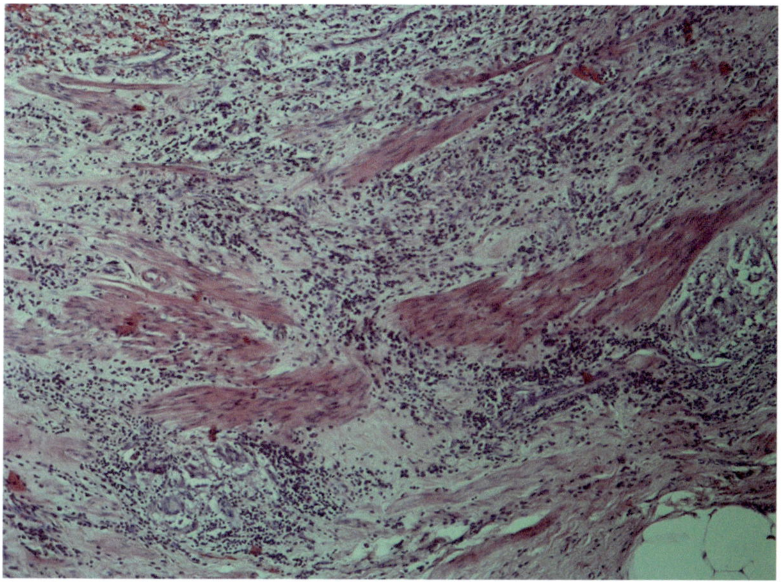

Fig. 3.8 TB of ureter. Granulomas in the wall of the ureter

estimate the value of endoscopy, bacteriology and histology for diagnosis BTB we analyzed 190 patients suspicious on BTB. All underwent X-ray examination, including intravenous urography and multispiral computer tomography, cystoscopy (excluding patients with cystostoma due to extremely low bladder volume), bladder biopsy. Patients with BTB 4 grade underwent cystectomy with iliocystoplastic, bladder tissue was also investigated. Bacteriology included luminescent microscopy of the sediment of urine, microscopy of smear colored by Zhiel-Nelsen technique, culture on three mediums, PCR-diagnostic, Bactec and GenExpert.

Among all 190 patients in 18 bladder tuberculosis (BTB) was confirmed, and in 172 – non-specific cystitis (NSC). Decreased volume was revealed in all BTB patients and in 15.7 % of NSC patients ($p<0.001$). Trabecules (66.7 %), ulcers (11.1 %), contact haemorrhages (83.8 %), bullous edema (44.4 %), and deformity of mouth of ureter (94.4 %) were found significantly more often in BTB patients. Hyperemia was met in BTB as often as in NSC (accordingly 38.9 % and 33.1 %).

Histology revealed specific TB inflammation in 11.8 % only, in other BTB patients lymphoid and eosinophilic infiltration as well as fibrosis prevailed. M. tuberculosis was found by culture in 11.1 %, by PCR – in 16.7 %, none – by microscopy.

There are no any endoscopic findings to confirm BTB, but there are some signs to suspect this disease. Histological and bacteriological confirmation is possible in 11.8 % only- mostly due to late examination, after long antibacterial therapy. So far as bladder TB is rarely confirmed by cystoscopy, bacteriology or histology, this

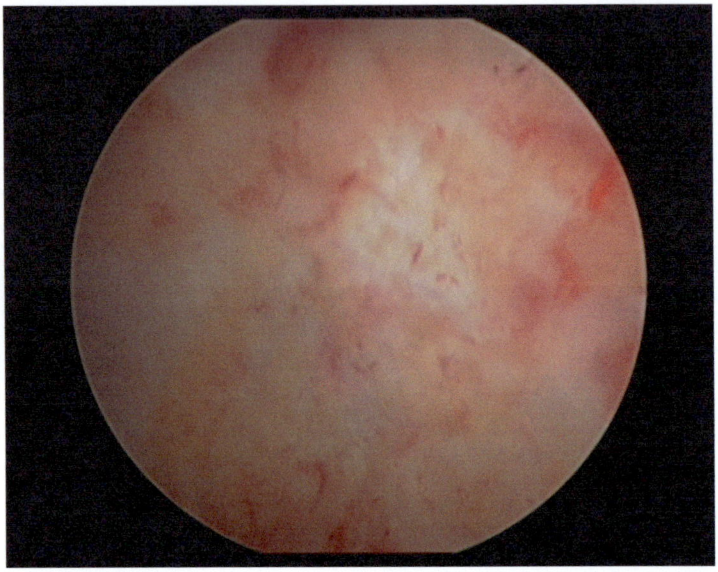

Fig. 3.9 Cystoscopy of the patient with confirmed bladder TB 2nd stage. Local hyperemia, edema

diagnosis may be established all patients with confirmed UGTB presenting dysuria and/or decreasing bladder volume.

Some cystoscopical pictures are shown on Figs 3.9, and 3.10.

The first two stages should be treated by standard anti-TB drugs, 3-rd stage – with standard anti-TB drugs and trospium chloride, and 4-th stage is indicated for cystectomy with following enteroplasty. Bladder TB is rather often complication of KTB, but its manifestation may be unusual and misguiding. Kumar et al. (1994) reported two cases of a TB cavity behind the bladder and prostate which initially eluded diagnosis, and were confirmed only after surgery. Typical for bladder TB situation was reported by Kaneko et al. (2008). A 24-year-old man experienced gross haematuria and dysuria several times a year from the age of 19, presenting to the Urological Department for the first time at age 21, when he was given standard antibiotic treatment for acute cystitis. We supposed, it was fluoroquinolone, which inhibit Mtb, but doesn't kill it for short course standard for UTI. Although urinary symptoms persisted, he failed to attend for follow-up. He attended another clinic at the age of 24 with increased urinary frequency. Transrectal ultrasonography revealed thickening of the bladder wall, concavity of the right bladder neck, and nodular changes extending from the left bladder neck to the left bladder wall, and Mtb was detected in the urine Kumar et al. (1994). For a long time bladder TB was overlooked – till it got stage 4 – incurable by anti-TB drug.

- **TB of urethra.** TB of the urethra is nowadays not a frequent complication; usually it is diagnosed at the stage of a stricture.

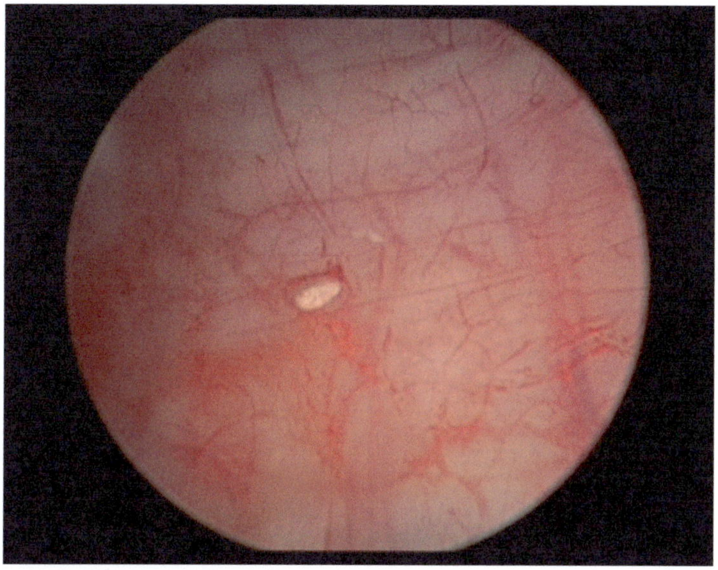

Fig. 3.10 Cystoscopy of the patient with confirmed bladder TB 2nd stage. Total hyperemia, full-blooded vessels, local edema, tubercle in the center

3.4.3 Clinical Features of Male Genital Tuberculosis (MGTB)

- **TB epididymitis** may be mono- bilateral; bilateral TB epididymitis is always secondary to prostate TB. Isolated TB epididymitis was found in 22 % as accidental surgical finding (Kulchavenya et al. 2012; Kulchavenya 2014).
- **TB of the testis** is always secondary to infection of the epididymis, which in most cases is blood-borne because of the extensive blood supply of the epididymis, particularly the lobus minor. In 62 % of patients with orchiepididymitis KTB is diagnosed as well. Every third patient has bilateral lesions. In about 12 % the disease is complicated by fistulas (Kulchavenya et al. 2012; Dell'Atti 2014). Every third patient has bilateral lesions. Isolated TB epididymitis was revealed in 22 % as accidental surgical finding. In about 12 % the disease is complicated by fistula (Kulchavenya et al. 2012). Fistulous form of TB orchiepididymitis is demonstrated on Fig 3.11.

Scrotal organs biopsy may be useful in the diagnosis of TB of external male genitals (Suárez-Grau et al. 2012). However, scrotal violation should be considered if the mass is malignant, and there were fatal complications after biopsies performed to non-treated patients with active UGTB due to fulminant generalization of TB. Both scrotal and prostate biopsies in patient with active TB may lead to fulminant generalization of TB with fatal outcome.

Nevertheless, diagnosis male genital tuberculosis is often incidental, based on histological investigation of the operational material after transurethral resection

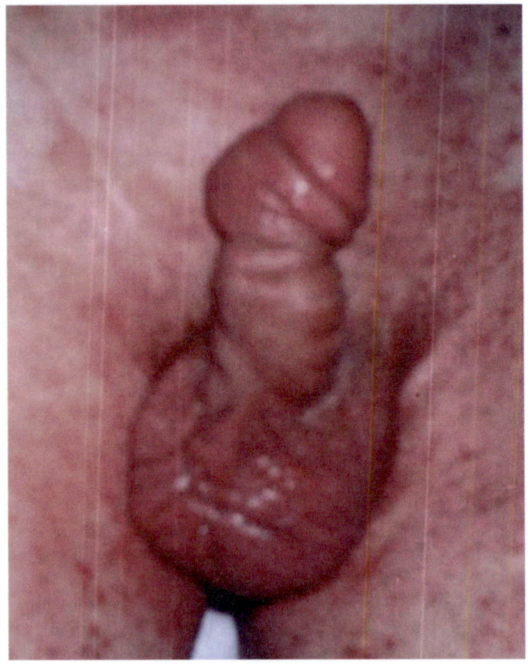

Fig. 3.11 TB orchiepididymitis, fistulous form

because of benign prostatic hyperplasia, of the biopsies, performed because of cancer was suspected etc. Pathohistology in all tissues may reveal caseous, fibrosis, granulomas (Figs. 3.12, 3.13, 3.14, 3.15, 3.16, 3.17, 3.18, and 3.19).

- **TB of the prostate** is an often under-diagnosed disease. Three quarters of men died from all forms of TB, had prostate TB, mostly overlooked alive (Kamyshan 2003), and every forth alive patients with pulmonary TB has prostate TB, confirmed by biopsy (Kulchavenya 2014). Prostate biopsy should be made only after urethrography for excluding caverns. Tissue of the gland should be investigated by histology and bacteriology, at least by PCR (Hemal et al. 2000; Singh et al. 2011).

  Prostate TB is important due to the following:

(a) It may also be a sexually transmitted disease. Up to 50 % of prostate TB patients have Mtb in their ejaculate if they are co-morbid with hepatitis and syphilis (Aphonin et al. 2006).
(b) It leads to infertility.
(c) It causes chronic pelvic pain like any other prostatitis, reducing significantly the quality of life (Kumar et al. 2015).
(d) It decreases the sexual function, also reducing the quality of life (Kulchavenya et al. 2012).

In 79 % prostate TB was accompanied by KTB, in 31 % by TB orchiepididymitis, and in 5 % isolated prostate TB was diagnosed (Kulchavenya et al. 2012). Kim

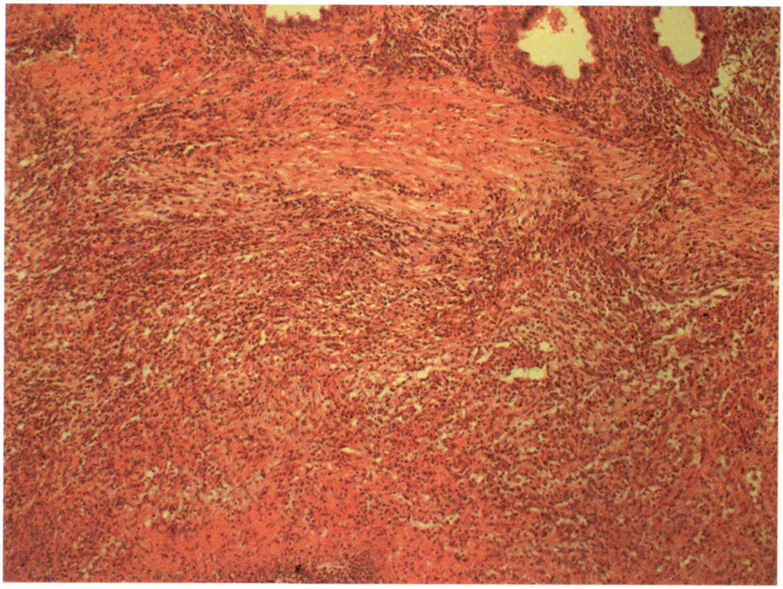

Fig. 3.12 TB of epididymis. Cellular repertoire of large granuloma wall: epithelioid cells, lymphocytes, fibroblasts. ×100. Hematoxylin and eosin

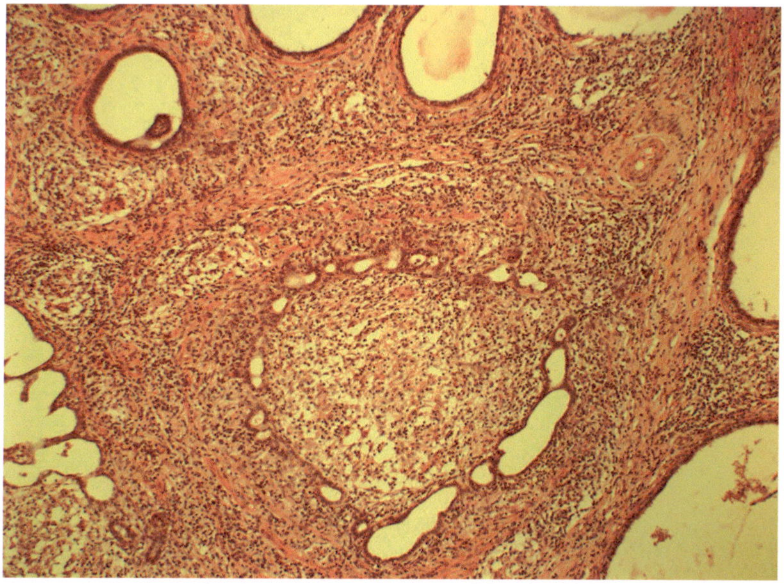

Fig. 3.13 TB of epididymis. Granulomatous inflammation without caseation. ×100. Hematoxylin and eosin

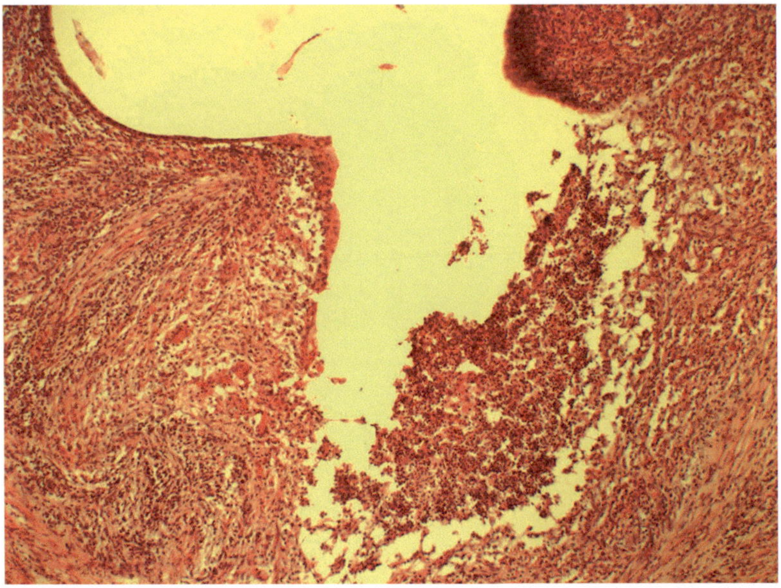

Fig. 3.14 TB of epididymis. Segment of tubular destruction, caused by granulomatous inflammatory infiltration. Forming caseous-lined cavity. ×100. Hematoxylin and eosin

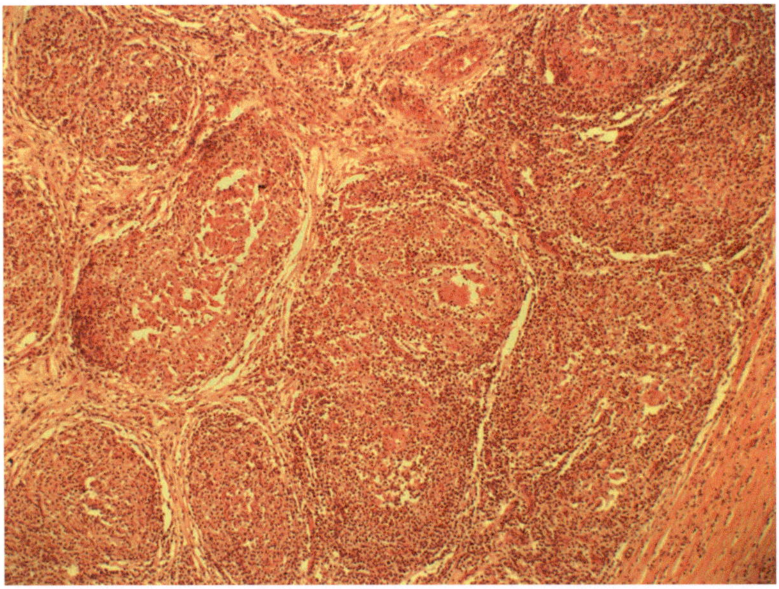

Fig. 3.15 TB granulomatous orchitis with displacement of glandular structures. Epithelioid granulomata of various size within stroma of testicle. ×100. Hematoxylin and eosin

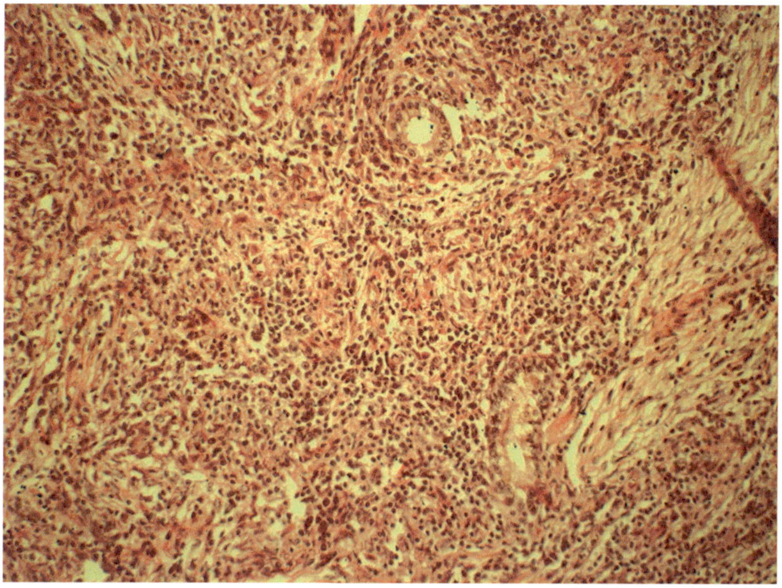

Fig. 3.16 TB granulomatous orchitis with displacement of glandular structures. ×200. van Gieson

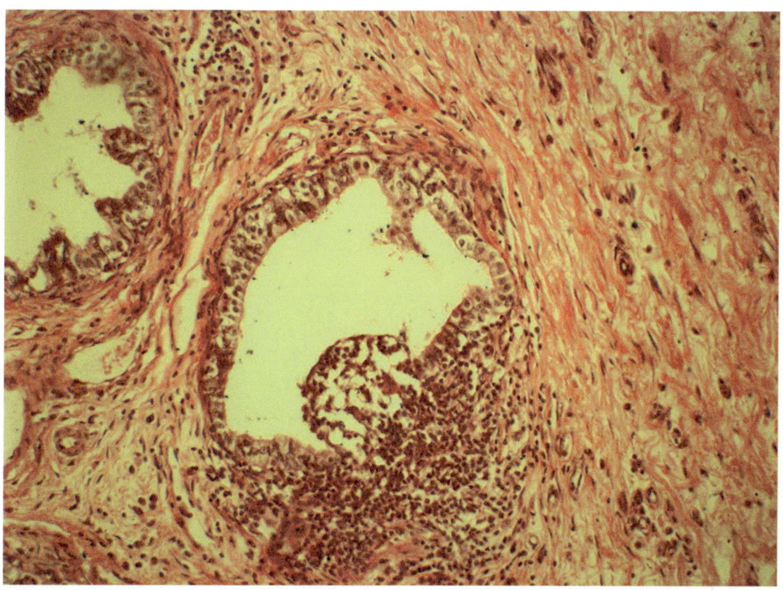

Fig. 3.17 TB of rete testis. Segmental granulomatous inflammation of ductulus efferens. ×200. van Gieson

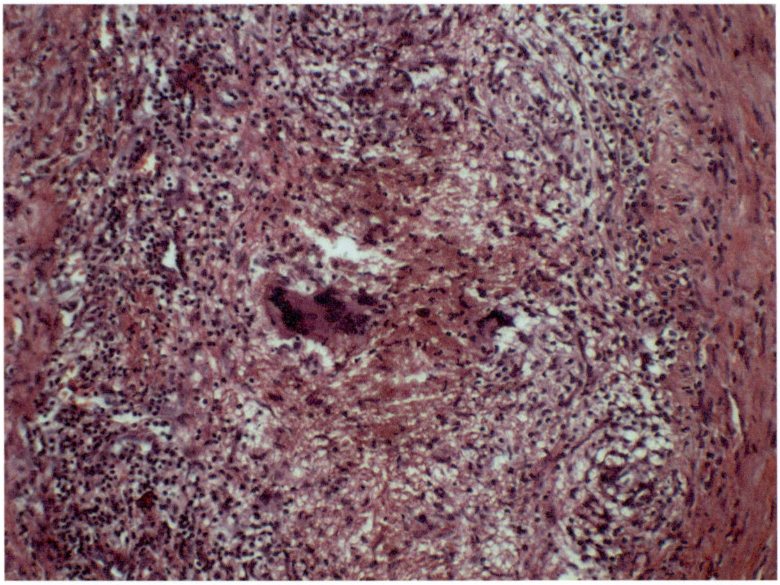

Fig. 3.18 TB of epididymis. Granulomatous inflammation with epithelioid and Langhans' giant cells. ×200. Hematoxylin and eosin

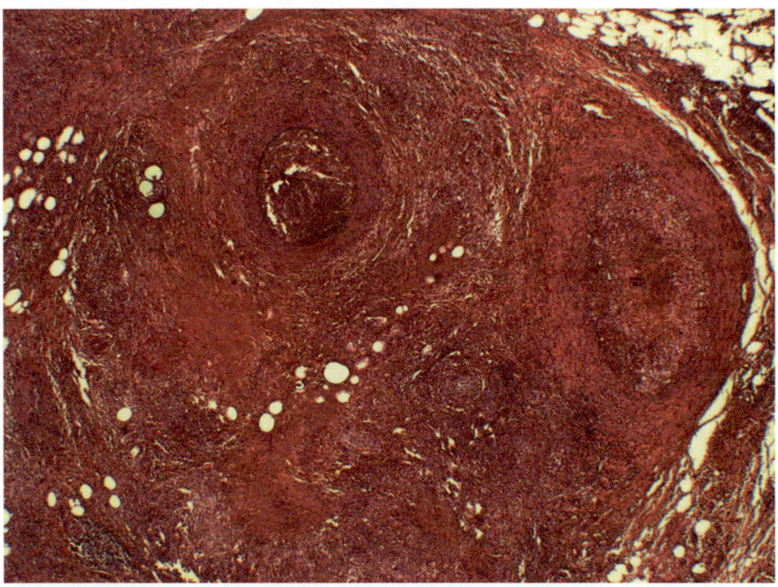

Fig. 3.19 TB of epididymis. Irregular fibrosis, mononuclear infiltration. ×40. Hematoxylin and eosin

et al. (2011) described a miliary tuberculosis as a complication of transrectal ultrasonography-guided prostate. A 75-year-old patient who presented with high fever and cough following TRUS-guided prostate biopsy for his high serum prostate-specific antigen (PSA) level (13.104 ng/ml) was diagnosed with miliary TB after clinical, laboratory, and radiological assessments. Histopathological examination of the prostate revealed TB with acid-fast bacilli. We would like to emphasize, that this patients at a glance had contra-indication for invasive procedure due to fever – actually he had miliary tuberculosis before prostate biopsy, not as a result of this operation.

Gupta et al. (2008) have found that prostate tuberculosis is uncommon and is usually found incidentally following transurethral resection – nevertheless there are no reports on transurethral resection for the surgery for BTB.

- **TB of seminal vesicles** is secondary to prostate TB and leads to infertility. As drainage of caseous ejaculate is difficult, TB of seminal vesicles exhibits a tendency to calcification (Stasinou et al. 2015).
- **TB of the penis** is very rare, but can occur after sexual intercourse with infected females (Narayana et al. 1976) or via a direct infection through a penile wound during ritual circumcision. Penile lesions present as ulcers on the glans or penile skin. Cutaneous penile TB in an HIV-positive man masquerading as a sexually transmitted infection was confirmed by positive cultures (Stockamp et al. 2013). Toledo-Pastrana et al. (2012) reported the case of a patient with ulcerous penile TB, presumably acquired through sexual intercourse. Kar and Kar (2012) have found primary TB of penis in a 31 years old male patient who presented with some ulcerated lesions on the glans penis. Diagnosis was established as primary tuberculosis of glans penis, confirmed by biopsy and supported by a strongly positive Mantoux test and positive TB-PCR. There was no co-existing tubercu-lous infection elsewhere.

Also Sah et al. (1999) revealed a 60-year-old man presented with multiple superficial ulcers on the glans penis. Histopathology, a positive tuberculin test result, and therapeutic response to antituberculous therapy confirmed the diagnosis of penile TB. Examination was otherwise normal except for a solitary enlarged reactive lymph node on the right side. And again there was no evidence of coexistent TB infection elsewhere.

Baskin and Mee (1989) reported a case of penis TB that presented as a subcutaneous nodule without superficial ulceration as well as Yonemura et al. (2004) who have experienced a case of penis TB that appeared as a scab on nodule. A 56-year-old man presented with a 4-month history of a painless subcutaneous nodule at the glans penis. Pathological findings of the nodule showed granulomatous inflammation. Tuberculin tests were strongly positive, but Mtb could not be detected. Savu et al. (2012) presented a case of penile tuberculosis with a bulky penoscrotal formation treated previously for the suspicion of Fournier gangrene. Nevertheless currently it is mainly a complication of BCG-therapy (Linden-Castro et al. 2014; Sharma et al. 2011; Chowdhury and Dey 2013).

References

Aphonin AB, Perezmanas EO, Toporkova EE, Khodakovsky EP (2006) Tuberculous infection as sexually transmitted infection. Vestnik poslediplomnogo obrazovaniya 3–4:69–71

Baskin LS, Mee S (1989) Tuberculosis of the penis presenting as a subcutaneous nodule. J Urol 141(6):1430–1431

Carrillo-Esper R, Moreno-Castañeda L, Hernández-Cruz AE, Aguilar-Zapata D (2010) A renal tuberculosis. Cir Cir 78(5):442–447

Chowdhury AR, Dey RK (2013) Penile tuberculosis following intravesical Bacille Calmette-Guérin immunotherapy. Indian J Urol 29(1):64–66. doi:10.4103/0970-1591.109989

Dell'Atti L (2014) Unusual isolated tubercolous epididymitis. Case report. G Chir 35(5–6):134–136

Figueiredo AA, Lucon AM (2008) Urogenital tuberculosis: update and review of 8961cases from the world literature. Rev Urol 10(3):207–217

Gupta N, Mandal AK, Singh SK (2008) Tuberculosis of the prostate and urethra: a review. Indian J Urol 24(3):388–391. doi:10.4103/0970-1591.42623

Hemal AK, Gupta NP, Rajeev TP, Kumar R, Dar L, Seth P (2000) Polymerase chain reaction in clinically suspected genitourinary tuberculosis: comparison with intravenous urography, bladder biopsy, and urine acid fast bacilli culture. Urology 56(4):570–574

Kamyshan IS (2003) Guideline on urogenital tuberculosis. Kuev 2003:363–424

Kaneko T, Kudoh S, Matsushita N, Kashiwabara Y, Tamura T, Yoshida I, Nomura K (2008) Case of bladder tuberculosis with onset at the age of nineteen--treatment of urinary tract tuberculosis in accordance with the new Japanese tuberculosis treatment guidelines. Nihon Hinyokika Gakkai Zasshi 99(1):29–34

Kar JK, Kar M (2012) Primary tuberculosis of the glans penis. J Assoc Physicians India 60:52–53

Kim CJ, Sano T, Takimoto K (2011) Miliary tuberculosis following transrectal ultrasonography (TRUS)-guided prostate biopsy. Korean J Urol 52(6):425–427. doi:10.4111/kju.2011.52.6.425. Epub 2011 Jun 17

Kulchavenya E (2010) Some aspects of urogenital tuberculosis. Int J Nephrol Urol 2(2):351–360

Kulchavenya E (2014) Urogenital tuberculosis: epidemiology, diagnosis, therapy. Springer, Cham/Heidelberg/New York/Dordrecht/London. doi:10.1007/978-3-319-04837-6, 137 p. ISBN 978-2-319-04836-9

Kulchavenya E, Kim CS, Bulanova O, Zhukova I (2012) Male genital tuberculosis: epidemiology and diagnostic. World J Urol 30(1):15–21. Epub 2011 May21. Review

Kumar A, Srivastava A, Mishra VK, Banerjee G (1994) Tubercular cavity behind the prostate and bladder: an unusual presentation of genitourinary tuberculosis. J Urol 151(5):1351–1352

Kumar S, Kashyapi BD, Bapat SS (2015) A rare presentation of tuberculous prostatic abscess in young patient. Int J Surg Case Rep 10:80–82. doi:10.1016/j.ijscr.2015.03.028. Epub 2015 Mar 18

Lenk S, Schroeder J (2001) Genitourinary tuberculosis. Curr Opin Urol 11(1):93–98

Linden-Castro E, Pelayo-Nieto M, Alias-Melgar A (2014) Penile tuberculosis after intravesical bacille Calmette-Guérin immunotherapy. Urology 84(2):e3. doi:10.1016/j.urology.2014.04.037. Epub 2014 Jun 21

Miyake H, Fujisawa M (2011) Tuberculosis in urogenital organs. Nihon Rinsho 69(8):1417–1421

Narayana AS, Kelly DG, Duff FA (1976) Tuberculosis of the penis. Br J Urol 48(4):274

Porter MF III (1894) Uro-Genital tuberculosis in the Male. Ann Surg 20(4):396–405

Sah SP, AshokRaj G, Joshi A (1999) Primary tuberculosis of the glans penis. Australas J Dermatol 40(2):106–107

Savu C, Surcel C, Mirvald C, Gîngu C, Hortopan M, Sinescu I (2012) Atypical primary tuberculosis mimicking an advanced penile cancer. Can we rely on preoperative assessment? Rom J Morphol Embryol 53(4):1103–1106

Sharma VK, Sethy PK, Dogra PN et al (2011) Primary tuberculosis of glans penis after intravesical Bacillus Calmette Guerin. Indian J Dermatol Venereol Leprol 77(1):47–50

Singh V, Sinha RJ, Sankhwar SN, Sinha SM (2011) Reconstructive surgery for tuberculous contracted bladder: experience of a center in northern India. Int Urol Nephrol 43(2):423–430

Stasinou T, Bourdoumis A, Owegie P, Kachrilas S, Buchholz N, Masood J (2015) Calcification of the vas deferens and seminal vesicles: a review. Can J Urol 22(1):7594–7598

Stockamp NW, Paul S, Sharma S, Libke RD, Boswell JS, Nassar NN (2013) Cutaneous tuberculosis of the penis in an HIV-infected adult. Int J STD AIDS 24:57–58. [Epub ahead of print]

Suárez-Grau JM, Bellido-Luque JA, Pastrana-Mejía A, Gómez-Menchero J, García-Moreno JL, Durán-Ferreras I, Guadalajara-Jurado JF (2012) Laparoscopic surgery of an enterovesical fistula of tuberculous origin (terminal ileum and sigmoid colon). Rev Esp Enferm Dig 104(7):391–392

Toledo-Pastrana T, Ferrándiz L, Pichardo AR, Muniaín Ezcurra MA, Camacho Martínez FM (2012) Tuberculosis: an unusual cause of genital ulcer. Sex Transm Dis 39(8):643–644. doi:10.1097/OLQ.0b013e318251577b

WHO (2014) Fact sheet N°104. Reviewed March 2014. Available on http://www.who.int/mediacentre/factsheets/fs104/en/

Wildbolz H (1937) Ueber urogenical tuberkulose. Schweiz Med Wochenschr 67:1125

Yonemura S, Fujikawa S, Su JS, Ohnishi T, Arima K, Sugimura Y (2004) Tuberculid of the penis with a scab on the nodule. Int J Uro 11(10):931–933

Chapter 4
Chemotherapy for Urogenital Tuberculosis

Abstract The first anti-tuberculosis drug *streptomycin* was created in 1945. Before this time the therapy for TB was based on diet and fresh air. Un-controlled using of antibiotics provoked development of drug resistant strains, so the history of urogenital TB can be divided into three periods: before antibiotics (AB), AB era and novo-days – MDR period. Mtb is drug-resistance, which may be: *mono* – Mtb are resistant to one of any antituberculous drugs; *poly* – Mtb are resistant to more than one of any drugs used for the treatment of the disease, excluding isoniazid and rifampicin simultaneously; *multi-drug resistance* (MDR) – Mtb are resistant to at least isoniazid and rifampicin, with or without resistance to other first-line drugs. Extensively drug-resistant TB (XDR-TB) refers to resistance to at least isoniazid and rifampicin, and to any fluoroquinolone, and to any of the three second-line injectables (amikacin, capreomycin and kanamycin). Persistence excluded an old specific for UGTB symptom – aseptic pyuria. Mtb hurts tissue and fades in persistence – for example, because the patient takes drugs for "UTI". Damaged tissues are rapidly colonized by E.Coli – and now co-morbidity of UGTB and non-specific UTI enriches 75 %.

WHO notes that five drugs are currently regarded as essential in the management of TB – isoniazid, rifampicin, pyrazinamide, streptomycin and ethambutol. Thioacetaxone is also widely used to supplement isoniazid in many developing countries because of its low cost. Other drugs, including para-aminosalicylic acid (PAS), kanamycin, cycloserine, capreomycin, viomycin and ethionamide, can be of value in treating patients with MDR, but, in general, are more expensive and more toxic.

Possibilities of chemotherapy may be limited by different side effects. Usually a patient with TB has at least one more disease, and co-morbidity demands to take into account potential drug interaction, which may lead both to increasing and decreasing therapeutic effect.

Keywords Urogenital tuberculosis • Therapy • Anti-tb drugs • Persistence • Resistence • Side effect

E. Kulchavenya, *Current Therapy and Surgery for Urogenital Tuberculosis*,
DOI 10.1007/978-3-319-28290-9_4

4.1 History (Before Antibacterial Era)

The millennial flight against tuberculosis has been characterized by several defeats. Roman physicians advised TB patients to consume better nutrition, take sea voyages and fresh air; during the Middle Ages, the 'royal touch' was considered as an effective remedy for TB scrofula. In the following centuries, TB was cured using old herbal preparations and new chemical compounds, mainly aimed at soothing symptoms; in addition, harmful approaches (for example, bleeding and purging) were commonly accepted, according to medical theories of that time (Riva 2014).

Because antibiotics were unknown, the only means of controlling the spread of infection was to isolate patients in private sanatoria or hospitals limited to patients with TB (Fig. 4.1).

In that period only a sanatorium regimen based on aerotherapy, bed rest, better nutrition, sunbathing and moderate physical exercise appeared to provide first partial successes. Some invasive approaches were also employed, such as lung collapse surgical interventions (for example, phrenicotomy, thoracoplasty) and artificial pneumothorax. And only when infectious agent of TB was discovered by Koch, attempts to destroy Mtb were undertook, but by using ineffective and sometimes harmful, dangerous preparation (Riva 2014).

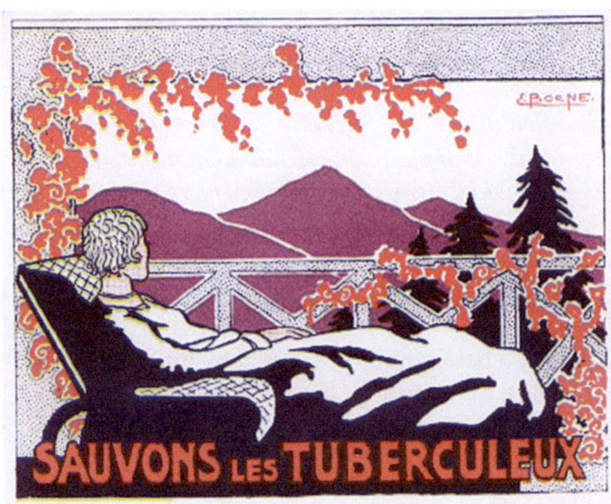

Fig. 4.1 Reproduction of color trade card, Paris, 1929 "Save the people with tuberculosis – romanticizing "consumption"". Association d'Hygiene Sociale et de Presentation Antituberculose du 1st Arr. Aon., Sauvons les Tuberculeux, color trade card

4.2 Antibacterial Era

In the second half of the past century a new antibacterial era started. The first anti-tuberculosis drug *streptomycin* was created by *Selman Abraham Waksman* in 1945. The development of anti-TB drugs (streptomycin, isoniazid, para-aminosalicylic acid, ethambutol and pyrazinamide) deeply revolutionized treatment for tuberculosis, allowing achievement of important successes. As an example I'd like to show the incidence rate of TB in the USSR and then in the Russian Federation (Fig. 4.2).

In the 1990's the incidence of TB decreased dramatically in Russia. The main reasons were: BCG-vaccination of newborns and creation of such antituberculous drugs as isoniazid, rifampicin, pyrazinamid, PASA, ethambutol, protionamid. Later the incidence increased till about 1990 (mostly because of social and economic factors) and remained stable for decade.

4.2.1 *MDR Period*

The history of urogenital TB can be divided into three periods: before antibiotics (AB), AB era and novo-days – MDR period.

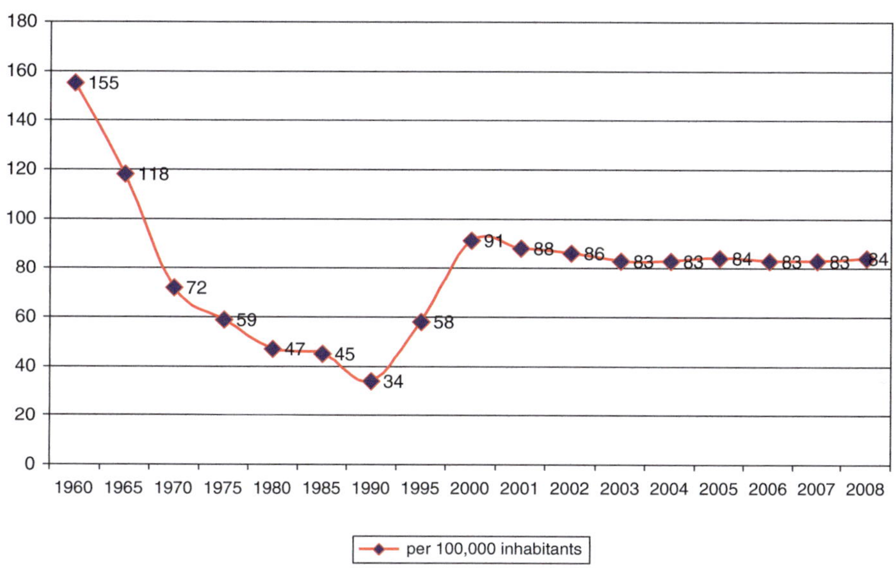

Fig. 4.2 Incidence of TB in the USSR (Russian Federation)

Before AB and in the beginning of the AB era, Mtb was calm and careless, it was confidents in her force, and it didn't put on her armour. At that time Mtb did not allow urine to be in any other microflora simultaneously. Once began, it continued to destroy a tissue up to full destruction.

In MDR period antibiotics significantly have changed a character of Mtb. Mtb had to put down her visor and to defend. Mtb can defend itself by two ways: by persistence and by resistance.

4.2.2 Persistence of Mtb

In bad, poor conditions (cold, heat, presence of antibiotics, even in low doses, insufficient of air etc.) Mtb doesn't multiply, hides in the cell and fades. Persistent Mtb is insensitive to the action of anti-bodies or antibiotic, which may kill her ONLY in a stage of her division. Normally Mtb replicates one time in 12–18 h, but in persistence it may rarely divide sporadically. A person infected with persistent Mtb has ***latent TB***. In a stage of persistence, ***self-recovery*** is possible due to apoptosis of infected cells. Mycobacteria can sleep, can lie dormant any length of time. If the immunity of macroorganism is strong, Mtb can remain in persistence lifelong. Accordingly a person over a lifetime will be infected, but will not be ill and will not be contagious.

Once (after colds, stress, intercurrent disease etc.) Mtb wakes up. When it has emerged from the darkness of persistence, Mtb is very aggressive, and progression of TB begins rapidly.

Persistence excluded the old specific for UGTB symptom – aseptic pyuria. Mtb hurts tissue and fades in persistence – for example, because a patient takes drugs for "UTI", masking UGTB – for example, fluoroquinolone, which inhibit Mtb, but doesn't kill it during a short course of the therapy for UTI. Damaged tissues are rapidly colonized by E.Coli – and now co-morbidity of UGTB and non-specific UTI enriches 75 %.

4.2.3 Resistance of Mtb

The second way of the defense of Mtb is drug-resistance, which may be:

- *mono* – Mtb are resistant to one of any antituberculous drugs;
- *poly* – Mtb are resistant to more than one of any drugs used for the treatment of the disease, excluding isoniazid and rifampicin simultaneously;
- *multi-drug resistance* (MDR) – Mtb are resistant to at least isoniazid and rifampicin, with or without resistance to other first-line drugs.
- *extensively drug-resistance* (XDR). Extensively drug-resistant TB (XDR-TB) refers to resistance to at least isoniazid and rifampicin, and to any fluoroquino-

lone, and to any of the three second-line injectables (amikacin, capreomycin and kanamycin).

About 450 000 people developed MDR-TB in the world in 2012. More than half of these cases were in India, China and the Russian Federation. It is estimated that about 9.6 % of MDR-TB cases had XDR-TB (WHO 2014). MDR and XDR TB are associated both with a higher incidence of treatment failures and of disease recurrence, as well as with higher mortality, than forms of TB sensitive to first-line drugs.

Reasons for development of drug resistant M. tuberculosis in UGTB patient are:

- Insufficient volume / duration of chemotherapy
- Peculiarities of TB process
- Condition of the patient and/or co-morbidity
- Non-optimal previous AB therapy for UTI.

More often drug-resistant mycobacteria are revealed in pulmonary TB patients. Compared with PTB, EPTB is negatively associated with multidrug resistance (OR 0.6) (Peto et al. 2009). Drug resistant Mtb were found in 79 % in pulmonary TB patients and only in 52 % in extrapulmonary TB patients (Vishnevskyi and Steklova 2008). There is no reasonable explanation of this fact, we must take it for what it is worth.

4.2.4 *How to Get Good Results in the Therapy for UGTB in MDR Period?*

Since 1995, over 56 million patients with pulmonary TB have been successfully treated and an estimated 22 million lives saved through use of DOTS and the Stop TB Strategy (WHO 2014). But there are some conditions for this benefit scenario:

1. The disease should be diagnosed on early stage (KTB 1–2);
2. The patient should be primary infected with sensitive Mtb;
3. The patient should be immunocompetent and shouldn't have any serious co-morbidity;
4. The regimen of the therapy should be optimal for good efficiency and prevention of the secondary drug resistance of Mtb;
5. The adherence of the patient to the therapy should be high.

Widespread, often un-controlling use of antibiotics significantly changed clinical features of UGTB, which hid under masks of another disease during 5.6 years on average before a correct diagnosis was made. We analyzed 816 history cases of UGTB patients to estimate clinical features and evaluate masks under which TB was hidden for a long time.

Most common complaints were flank pain (68 %), dysuria (48 %) and renal colic (24 %); among laboratory signs – pyuria (78 %) and haematuria (34 %). Patients were treated by urologists or GPs with misdiagnoses of pyelonephritis (27 %), cystitis (43 %), cancer (8 %) or urolithiasis (22 %) during 5.6 years on average. Positive smear was in 17 % and positive culture of Mtb was in 44 %. Sixty four percent were diagnosed in late complicated cavernous stage, when surgery is necessary – and 90 % of operations were nephrectomy due to total involvement of kidney tissue.

Hence most common masks of UGTB are pyelonephritis, cystitis and urolithiasis. UGTB presents non-specific symptoms and laboratory findings, except for positive Mtb culture, but only about 44 % of cases are culture-positive. This is one of the main reasons for late and poor diagnosis of UGTB. The significance of UGTB may be considerable when the high prevalence of overall TB and the asymptomatic nature of UGTB are taken into account.

We analyzed the histories of 167 patients with renal TB. About 7 % of them had acute onset, were operated on in clinics of general urology and their previous therapy didn't matter. Ninety three percent had chronic disease misdiagnosed as UTI, and for a long time they were treated with antibiotics, mostly for "cystitis". Among them only in about 40 % were the so-called "small forms" of kidney TB diagnosed – TB of renal parenchyma and TB papillitis. Eighty percent of these patients received optimal antibiotics, which don't inhibit Mtb (fosfomycin, gentamycin, nitrofurantoin, cephalosporins). Insufficient effect of the therapy allowed suspicion of TB, and a correct diagnosis was soon established. Then another 62 % of patients were revealed too late, with caverns – because in 75 % they were treated non-optimal, with antibiotics, which Mtb (fluoroquinolones, amycacin) and compels her to hide in persistence. And please let me remind the reader: if not treated, a person with TB infects an average of 10 to 15 new people each year, and TB is a sexually transmitted disease and one of the common reasons for both male and female infertility.

4.2.5 *How to Improve an Adherence and Compliance*

It is not secret – a poverty-ridden and asocial person is more liable to have any disease, including TB. These patients have a low motivation to undertake a long-time unpleasant treatment and put some limitation on fighting the disease. Poor adherence to Tb treatment is one of the main challenges for TB control, as it fosters TB transmission in the community and leads to drug resistance (Mirtskhulaya et al. 2013).

How can we improve the adherence? It was shown that additional food supplements improve adherences for care and treatment for TB patients, support treatment and minimize drug side effects together with results of the therapy (Kombe and Kapalata 2013; Kisonga et al. 2013). If rifampicin provokes an adverse effect, it can be replaced by rifabutin with the same efficiency but better tolerance (Chien et al. 2013).

One more reason for low adherence may be insufficient knowledge of both physicians and patients on fatal danger of TB for a patient, his family and society as a whole. It has resulted in interruption of the therapy and loss to follow-up – so called "default" (van der Werf et al 2013). TB treatment default rate remains above 10 % globally (Mirtskhulaya et al. 2013). Claasens et al (2013) reported, that in South Africa 25 % of new-revealed TB patients did not start treatment in a timely manner at primary healthcare facilities. These patients, defined as "initially lost to follow up" may transit Mtb within communities thereby contributing to the epidemic.

Mirtskhulaya et al. (2013) have found that the rate of defaulting was higher during the initial 3 months of chemotherapy. Multiple factors were attributed by defaulting patients as a cause for abandoning treatment, whereas different factors were independently associated with the TB therapy default. Authors believe that strengthening of outpatient treatment and enhanced psycho-social support to TB patients may reduce default rates.

Patients also used to interrupt the treatment because of side effects of anti-TB drugs (Chepuri Nagaraj et al. 2013).

4.2.6 *How Can We Prevent Drug Resistance and Improve Results of the Therapy for UGTB?*

TB is a treatable and curable disease. Active, drug-sensitive TB disease is treated with a standard 6-month course of four antimicrobial drugs that are provided with information, supervision and support to the patient by a health worker or trained volunteer. Without such supervision and support, treatment adherence can be difficult and the disease can spread. The vast majority of TB cases can be cured when medicines are provided and taken properly.

We prevent drug resistance and improve results of the therapy for UGTB by:

- Early diagnostic.
- Optimization chemotherapy.
- Using pathogenetic therapy.

Poor knowledge of the doctors and the population, absence of the specific features, non-optimal antibacterial therapy for non-specific UTI resulted in late diagnosis of UGTB with polycavernous complicated forms typical picture is shown in Fig. 4.3.

Late-diagnosed complicated form of cavernous UGTB (Fig. 4.4) can't be cured by chemotherapy at all, surgery (often radical) is necessary.

And KTB 1–2 stages without complications can be healed easyily and quickly.

4.2.7 *Tuberculosis and Cancer*

Even if the TB-patient is cured, he doesn't become absolutely healthy; more or less sequels remain. Mor et al (2013) estimated long-term mortality and causes of death among patients who recovered from TB. Authors have found that these patients are at higher risk of mortality compared with the general population adjusted for age and sex, mainly in males and in the ages of 24–55. The overall most common diagnosis was malignancy.

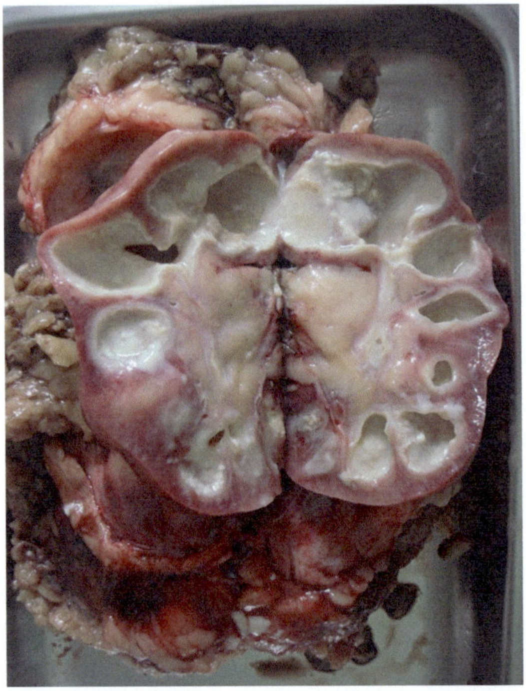

Fig. 4.3 Late-diagnosed kidney TB 4th stage – polycavernous kidney TB – operational material

Prostate cancer is one of the most common types of cancer and it is the second commonest cause of cancer-related death among men in the western world. Silberstein et al. (2013) have found microscopic prostate cancer in up to 30 % of men between 20–40 years old . In Japan, of 115,881 men attending the prostate cancer screening, 6099 men needed a second screening. Overall, 2320 of 6099 patients screened a second time underwent prostate biopsy, and 1073 men of them were diagnosed with prostate cancer (Koizumi et al. 2014).

Provocative factors for prostate cancer are unknown exactly. A recent study showed that chronic prostate inflammation accelerates prostate cancer progression (Simons et al. 2015), promotes initiation of diverse malignancies, enhances basal-to-luminal differentiation, and accelerates initiation of prostate cancer originating from basal cells (Kwon et al. 2014; Liu and Goldstein 2014; Sandhu 2008).

TB is a very chronic disease, so hyperchronic TB inflammation may provoke a malignization. Thus, TB may predispose a cancer, and prostate TB and prostate cancer have about the same clinical features, and the doctor has to have a highly suspicious index to recognize concomitant diseases. It is underlined by the following case history of our patient.

Case Report A 72 years old man was presented to our Institute in March 2011 with complaints of frequency and urgency, weakening urine stream, night sweats, bladder and perineal pain. In 1987 the patient had had a pulmonary TB and had been treated during 10 months with three anti-TB drugs (isoniazid, rifampicin, and strep-

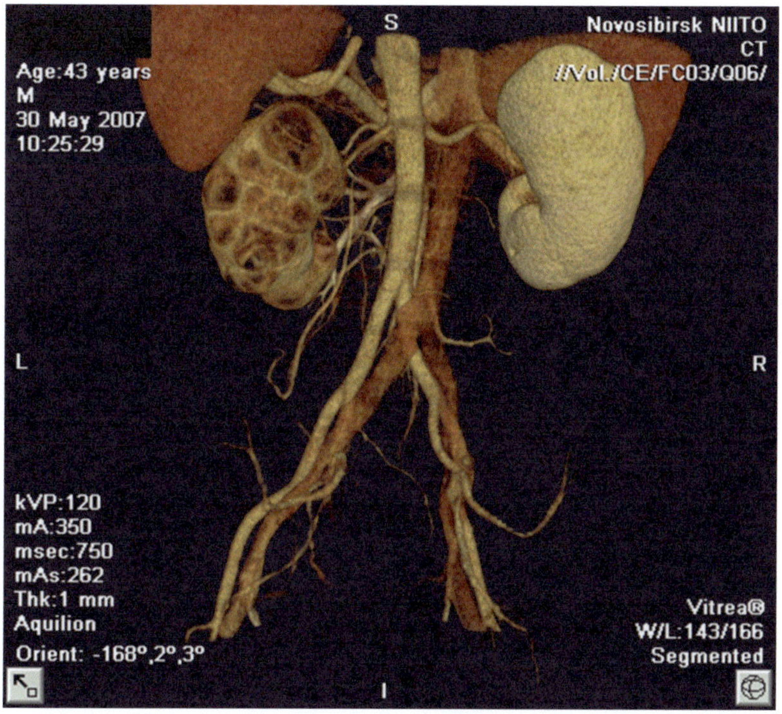

Fig. 4.4 Slice –tomogram: late-diagnosed kidney TB 4th stage – polycavernous kidney TB

tomycin) with good result. In 1990 the patient presented with hemospermia, strong perineal pain and was referred to a TB-urologist. Full examination revealed pyospermia, hemospermia and caverns of the prostate. Growth of Mtb was found both in ejaculate and prostate secretion. Mtb was sensitive to all anti-TB drugs. The pulmonary TB was not reactivated. The patient was treated during 10 months with four anti-TB drugs (isoniazid, rifampicin, streptomycin and pyrazinamide) again with good efficacy: pain and hemospermia disappeared and pyospermia decreased significantly. The prostate caverns, however, remained as complete healing of prostate tissue destructions is not possible. In 1993 the patient complained again of dysuria, perineal pain, and painful ejaculation. A relapse of prostate TB was finally diagnosed. Mtb did not grow, but could be detected in the ejaculate by polymerase chain reaction (PCR). The pulmonary TB remained inactive. The patient received isoniazid, rifampicin, streptomycin, PAS and pyrazinamid for 4 months, than isoniazid and rifampicin only for the rest of the year and in addition tocopherol, thiamin, phytotherapy, dimexid, and non-steroid inflammatory drugs. The patient also received rehabilitation courses annually for 5 years in a special anti-TB sanatorium. The patient was healed and remained well until March 2011, when pain and dysuria appeared again. Pyospermia with growth of *Enterobacter sp.* in prostatic secretion was found, but Mtb was not detected by any method. X-ray examination showed huge caverns of the prostate with calcification (Fig. 4.5).

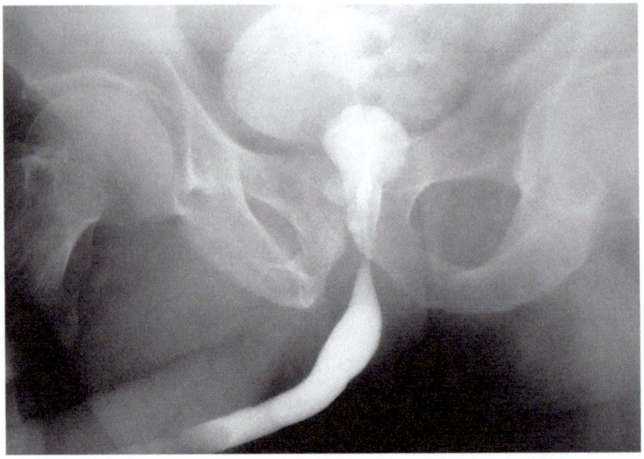

Fig. 4.5 Urethrogram: cavern of the prostate with calcification

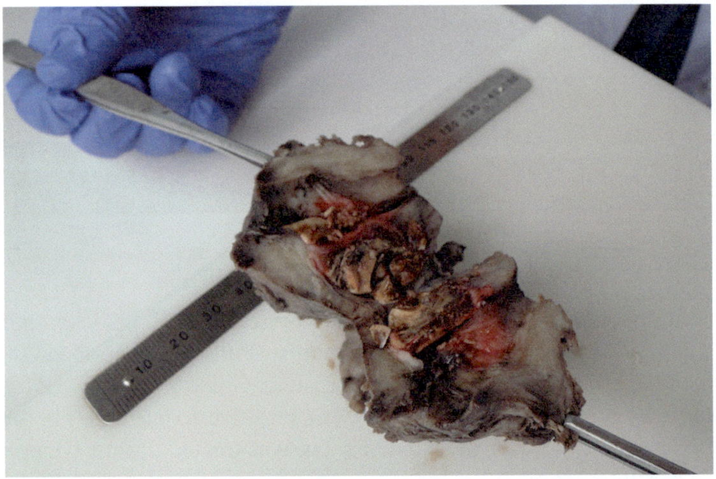

Fig. 4.6 Cured cavernous prostate tuberculosis with calcified caseation and secondary prostate cancer

As the PSA level was 11 ng/ml, prostate biopsy was performed and a solid-glandular cancer was found by histological examination. There was, however, no active TB inflammation in the biopsies. The patient underwent radical prostatectomy. The section of the prostate gland revealed huge TB caverns filled with stones (actually calcified caseation) as demonstrated in Fig. 4.6.

Histo-pathohistological investigations revealed a proliferation of the glandular prostate cancer with invasion of the capsule in the right and left lobes. The cavity walls of the caverns were lined with transitional epithelium with dense calcium salts in the lumen. In the seminal vesicles glandular tumor structures were growing into the muscle layer. Active TB inflammation was not found.

Although male genital TB seems to be a rare disease, 77 % of men who died from TB of all localizations had prostate TB, mostly overlooked during their lifetimes (Kulchavenya and Krasnov 2010). In a recent study 93 patients suspicious of prostate TB underwent ultrasound guided core prostate biopsy. Probes were investigated by PCR, pathomorphology and culture. Mtb was found by PCR in10.7 %, but Mtb culture was only positive in 6.9 %. Patho-histology revealed inflammation in 94.6 % of probes, fibrosis in 65.6 %, intraprostatic neoplasia in 9.7 %, cancer in 5.4 %, and TB in 24.7 % (Kulchavenya and Krasnov 2010).

Thus, prostate TB is rather often diseases, and all such patients have heightened risk of the development of prostate cancer.

UGTB is difficult to be diagnosed, and cancer is one of the most frequent diagnostic errors. Kho and Chan (2012) reported about a 20-year-old man who presented with a slow-growing painless scrotal tumor for 2 months, initially suspicious for a right paratesticular tumor. The patient underwent operation and patho-histology revealed TB.

Another case history was described by López Barón et al. (2009). A 65 year old man presented with symptoms of frequency, dysuria and weight loss within the last 6 months, without pulmonary symptoms and negative ELISA test for HIV. Digital rectal examination revealed a high volume, irregular and hard prostatic gland. Ultrasound investigation showed a prostatic volume of 39 cm^3, without sign of malignancy. The prostate biopsy showed multiple granulomas and the Zhiel-Neelsen staining was positive for Mtb.

Thus, UGTB should be considered as differential diagnosis for both, neoplastic and infectious–inflammatory diseases. UGTB mimics often even of cancer. An incorrect diagnosis leads to unnecessary surgical intervention, as UGTB should be treated by drugs only, at least if it has been diagnosed in time. Prostate TB like any other chronic infectious inflammation may predispose for prostate cancer. In any case high PSA levels are an indication for prostate biopsy, especially if the patient has a long-term history of an infectious-inflammatory process in the prostate.

4.2.8 Antituberculous Drugs

WHO notes that five drugs are currently regarded as essential in the management of TB – isoniazid, rifampicin, pyrazinamide, streptomycin and ethambutol. Thioacetaxone is also widely used to supplement isoniazid in many developing countries because of its low cost. Other drugs, including para-aminosalicylic acid (PAS), kanamycin, cycloserine, capreomycin, viomycin and ethionamide, can be of value in treating patients with MDR, but, in general, are more expensive and more toxic.

The classification of anti-TB drugs is given in the Table 4.1.

An ideal anti-TB drug, apart from being cheap and of low toxicity, would consequently need to posses:

1. Potent bactericidal activity against metabolically active bacilli;

Table 4.1 The classification of the anti-TB drugs

Essential First line anti-TB drugs (basic)	Second line anti-TB drugs (reserve)	Third line drugs for special clinical situation
Isoniazid (H)	Protionamyde (Pt)/ Ethionamyde (Et)	Amoxicillin/Clavulanate
Rifampicin (R)	Kanamycin (K)	Meropenem
Pyrazinamide (Z)	Amikacin (A)	Imipenem
Streptomycin (S)	Capreomycin (Cap)	Clarithromycin
Ethambutol (E)	Cycloserin (Cs)	Linezolid
	Rifabutin (Rb)	
	Para-Aminosalicylic Acid (PAS)	
	Fluoroquinolones (Fq)	
	Bedaquilin (Bq)	
	Perhlozone (Pz)	
	Terizidon (Tz)	

Table 4.2 Groups of second-line anti-tuberculosis agent

Group name	Anti-TB agent	Abbreviation
2nd line parenteral agents	Kanamycin	Km
	Amicacin	Amk
	capreomycin	Cm
Fluoroquinolones	Levofloxacin	Lfx
	Moxifloxacin	Mfx
	Gatifloxacin	Gfx
	Ofloxacin	Ofx
Oral bacteriostatic 2nd line anti-TB drugs	Ethionamyde	Eto
	Protionamyde	Pto
	Para-aminisalycilic acid	PAS
	Cycloserine	Cs
	Terizidone	Trd
Group 5 drugs	Clofazimine	Cfz
	Linezolid	Lzd
	Amoxicillin/clavulonat	Amx/Clv
	Thioacetazone	Thr
	Clarithromycin	Clr
	Imipenem	Imp

2. Potent sterilizing activity against semidormant persisting bacilli; and
3. Potential to prevent the emergence of resistant organism throughout the period of chemotherapy (WHO 1991).

For the therapy of MDR-TB patients WHO offers special classification of anti-TB drugs (Table 4.2).

Table 4.3 Properties of the essential anti-TB drugs

Drug	Drug property	Target bacilli	Site of an action	Eligible for UGTB
Isoniazid	Bactericidal after 24 h. High potency: kills >90 % active Mtb in first few days of treatment	Rapid and intermediate growing bacilli	Intracellular and extracellular	High recommended
Rifampicin	Bactericidal within 1 h. High potency. Most effective sterilising agent	All populations including dormant bacilli	Intracellular and extracellular	High recommended
Pyrazinamide	Bactericidal with a low potency. Achieves its sterilising action within 2–3 months	Slow growing bacilli	Intracellular bacilli only (macrophages)	High recommended
Ethambutol	Low potency. Minimises the emergence of drug resistance. Bacteriostatic	All bacterial populations	Intracellular and extracellular	Not recommended
Streptomycin	Bactericidal with a low potency	Rapidly growing bacilli	Extracellular	Not recommended

NB. Other drugs not generally considered as second-line anti-tuberculosis agents were also used to treat drug-resistant TB in some of the cohorts included in this analysis. These included the parenteral agent *viomycin,* the fluoroquinolones *ciprofloxacin* and *sparfloxacin,* as well as *azithromycin, roxithromycin, high-dose isoniazid* and *thioridazine,* which were included under the Group 5.

Below in the Table 4.3 the characteristic of essential drugs is given.

Isoniazid, which decimates the bacillary population within a few days of starting treatment, is unrivalled in its bactericidal potency – and it fairly is estimated as main anti-TB drug. Rifampicin and ethambutol have moderate bactericidal activity, while streptomycin, pyrazinamide and thioacetazone have little or no bactericidal action (Mitchison 2003).

4.2.8.1 Genetically Determined Metabolism of Isoniazid

One of the putative reasons of the low efficiency of anti-TB therapy may be fast metabolism of isoniazid. All people may be divided into three classes: fast, intermediate and slow inactivators of isoniazid. Concentration of acetyl-isoniazid and hydrazine-isoniazid was investigated in TB patients with consideration of their acetylation genotype by Kresyun et al. (2013). The authors concluded that the frequency of hepatotoxicity may depend on acetylation genotype. It is clear that results of the chemotherapy depends on the acetylation genotype too – but only if the patient receives the drug per os, intravenous administration levels these differences.

4.2.8.2 Isoniazid and Pyridoxine

Isoniazid is associated with pyridoxine deficiency because it interferes competitively with pyridoxine metabolism by inhibiting the formation of the active form of the vitamin B6, and hence often results in peripheral neuropathy. Nevertheless it is a great mistake to prescribe isoniazid and pyridoxine simultaneously – in fact they are antagonist, and if the patient takes isoniazid and pyridoxine together – he reduces a dose of isoniazid. Of course, combined administration increases tolerance, but decreases efficiency. If the patient has an indication for vitamin B6 (for example, because of neuropathy), pyridoxine should be administered separately from isoniazid, in 4–6 h during a meal.

4.2.8.3 New Drugs and New Forms of Old Drugs as a Method to Improve the Efficiency of the Therapy

There were many attempts to create a better form of anti-TB drugs. Nanocomposites of PAS with Zn/Al LDH and with ZLH were found to possess strong antimycobacterial and antimicrobial properties. In addition, these formulations were found to be highly biocompatible: about 80 % cell viability against normal human lung cells (which are the cells that most commonly reside in the place of *M. tuberculosis*) and mouse fibroblast cells (a standard cell line used in cytotoxicity studies) (Saifullah et al. 2014). The recent study describes the development of an antituberculosis nanodelivery formulation based on para-aminosalicylic acid with zinc layered hydroxides using $ZnNO_3$ salt as a precursor. The PAS *in vitro* efficacy was found to be fourfold better when used in the developed formulation compared to the free drug PAS (Saifullah et al. 2014).

Insufficient results of the anti-TB treatment dictate a necessity of the creation new drugs or new forms of the drugs. These drugs should have enhanced bioavailability, the ability to get exactly TB zone, to provide a prolonged effect, thereby reducing the number of intakes and risk of side effects. In the Russian Federation the preclinical comparative study of anti-TB activity and toxicity of nano-rifampicin, nano-levofloxacin and nano-cycloserin with substances of these drugs in their original form was carried out (Erokhin et al. 2013). The authors have showed a superiority of nano-drugs in mice.

Also old well-known in general practice medications surprisingly may demonstrate anti-TB activity. For example, clofazimine – it was first approved by the Food and Drug administration in 1986 for treatment of leprosy. Although clofazimine has shown activity against Mtb (including drug-resistant strains) in vitro and in animal studies, it has not been approved for use in TB therapy. Clofazimine fell out of favour due to its lower efficacy but has gained renewed interest as the range of available drugs for the therapy for drug-resistant TB is limited. Efficiency of the clofazimine in MDR-TB patients was evaluated in multicenter, randomized controlled study. It was proved that using clofazimine to treat MDR-TB can significantly improve clinical symptoms, promote cavity closure, and accelerate sputum negative conversion. Also in the group treated with clofazimine, improvements of life quality and good drug tolerance were noted (Tang et al. 2013a). Shean et al (2013) noted good tolerance of clofazimine: prevalence of side effects was very low. Authors consider clofazimine as potentially useful drug for inclusion on regimens for XDR-TB patients.

Massive neutrophilic infiltration is TB nature, so inflammation might be a key factor in the progression towards active tuberculosis. Vilaplana and Cardona (2013) asked themselves: “Could the common anti-inflammatories be the new coadjuvant treatment against tuberculosis?”, and trying to discern the transformation of latent TB into cavernous form discovered ibuprofen as a clue treatment and prevention against TB.

Tang et al. (2013b) estimated efficiency of linezolid in complex therapy for extremely drug-resistant (XDR) TB patients. Linezolod is a new antibiotic with activity against Mtb in vitro and in animal studies. Linezolod containing chemotherapy for treatment of XDR-TB may significantly promote cavity closure, accelerate sputum culture conversion and improve treatment success rates. Meanwhile side effects might be tolerated and resolve after suitable intervention.

Aminoglycosides (AGs) are considered a critical component on MDR-TB treatment regimens. The question is – effectiveness and toxicity of aminoglycosides: a matter of dead or deaf? Modongo et al (2013) analyzed 410 MDR-TB patients who were treated with AGs. 80 % had good clinical outcomes and 68 % developed ototoxicity.

Normally fluoroquinolones are contraindicated for children under 14, but so severe infection as TB forces to neglect potential risk for the recovery from the disease, even with sequels.

An eternal question in anti-TB therapy, mentioned above is a matter of dead or complications? Thee et al (2013) used ofloxacin and levofloxacin in 23 children (among them three had alongside with TB an HIV-infection). Children seem to eliminate ofloxacin and levofloxacin faster than adults, leading to a drug exposure about half of that in adults following a standard oral dose (ofloxacin 800 mg and levofloxacin 750 mg). Higher or twice daily dosing of ofloxacin and levofloxacin might be needed to provide compatible exposures associated with clinical efficiency in adults. No QT prolongation occurred.

Because of standard therapy demonstrates rather low efficiency, many new regimens are created and tested. So, it was proved by randomized study, that a 6-month regimen with weekly 1200 mg rifapentine and moxifloxacin in the continuation phase was non-inferior to the control, even at the 95 % level. This regimen was safe and well tolerated. But the 4-month course was inferior to the control (Jindani et al. 2013).

After decades of quiescence in the development of antituberculosis medications, bedaquiline and delamanid have been conditionally approved for the treatment of drug-resistant tuberculosis, while several other novel compounds (AZD5847, PA-824, SQ109 and sutezolid) have been evaluated in phase II clinical trials (Olaru et al. 2014). bedaquiline (Sirturo) and delamanid (Deltyba) were authorised by the European Medicines Agency under its 'conditional market authorisation' scheme for use as part of an appropriate combination regimen for pulmonary MDR-TB in adult patients "when an effective treatment regimen cannot otherwise be composed for reasons of resistance or tolerability".

Bedaquiline is the first drug of a new class approved for the treatment of TB in decades. Bedaquiline is metabolized by cytochrome P450 (CYP) 3A4 to a less-active M2 metabolite. Its terminal half-life is extremely long (5–6 months), complicating evaluations of drug-drug interactions. Rifampicin and rifapentine, two anti-TB drugs now being optimized to shorten TB treatment duration, are potent inducers of CYP3A4 (Svensson et al. 2014). Rifamycin reduce bedaquiline concentrations substantially. In line with current treatment guidelines for drug-susceptible TB, concomitant use is not recommended, even with dose adjustment (Svensson et al. 2014).

Delamanid (Deltyba(®)), a nitroimidazo-oxazole derivative, is a new anti-tuberculosis (TB) drug which exhibits potent in vitro and in vivo antitubercular activity against drug-susceptible and -resistant strains of Mycobacterium tuberculosis. It is approved in several countries, including Japan and those of the EU, for use as part of an appropriate combination regimen in adults with multidrug-resistant tuberculosis (MDR-TB) when an effective treatment regimen cannot otherwise be composed due to resistance or tolerability (Blair and Scott 2015).

There is no enough experience on using these drugs in pulmonary TB patients and there is no experience at all on using these drugs in extrapulmonary TB patients, including urogenital.

Pharmaceutical Industries offer us only combination of old drugs, often in non-optimal doses. In 1965-th the possibility of chemotherapy for TB was fresh and strong like this lemon, today this possibility is poor, and what will be tomorrow?

4.3 Adverse Effect of Chemotherapy for UGTB

Possibilities of chemotherapy may be limited by different side effects. Usually a patient with TB has at least one more disease, and co-morbidity demands to take into account potential drug interaction, which may lead both to increasing and decreasing therapeutic effect.

High incidence of liver toxicity induced by pyrazinamide, rifampicin, isoniazid was revealed. The risk factors of drug-induced hepatitis so far reported included elderly, positive hepatitis C virus antibody, low serum albumin and so on (Grosset et al. 2012). Liver injury was characterized as being mild and moderate and the type of injury associated was represented by pure cholestasis and hepatocanalicular lesions. Probably, rifampicin is the drug responsible for this kind of evolution aggravating the hepatotoxicity induces by isoniazid and pyrazinamide (Mitchison and Davies 2012). Liver injury was characterized as being mild and moderate and the type of injury associated was represented by pure cholestasis and hepatocanalicular lesions (Kolpakova et al. 2001). Probably, rifampicin is the drug responsible for this kind of evolution aggravating the hepatotoxicity induces by isoniazid and pyrazinamide. Isoniazid and pyrazinamide are both well-known hepatotoxic drugs. When isoniazid is used, the hepatic lesion appears before than when pyrazinamide is used (de Souza et al. 1996).

Drug resistance was noted in 40.1 % of patients with renal TB. Pyrazinamide, streptomycin, and ethambutol were most toxic to these patients. There was a higher likelihood of drug intolerance in females with bilateral nephrotuberculosis complicated by chronic renal failure (Kul'chavenia and Kuznetsov 1998; Shutskaia et al. 1991).

The profile of patients treated by DOTS scheme and presenting with adverse reactions showed that the majority of patients (53 %) had gastrointestinal reactions, the commonest presenting complaint being nausea and vomiting. General aches and pains were complained by about 35 % and giddiness was the presenting complaint in 27 % irrespective of the use of streptomycin. Skin rash and itching was complained by about 17 % of patients and 11 % complained of arthralgia, while only 1 % had hepatotoxicity during treatment. Majority of the adverse reactions (67 %) were observed within the first four weeks of treatment (Pereira et al. 2000; Dhingra et al. 2004; Zierski and Bek 1980).

Layer and Engelhardm (1986) described a case lupus erythematosus (SLE) and concomitant pulmonary tuberculosis in a 46-year-old female patient. In the course of the tuberculostatic therapy, there occurred six episodes of exacerbation of drug-induced SLE signs and symptoms including fever, myalgia, swelling of joints, butterfly rash and high titers of antinuclear antibodies. These exacerbations were induced by single-agent or combination therapy with ethambutol, pyrazinamide, streptomycin and/or prothionamide and resolved readily after discontinuation of the drug(s).

Isoniazid-induced lupus erythematosus affects either sex equally and the most common presenting feature is arthralgia or arthritis with anemia. Fever and pleuritis occur in approximately half of the cases, and pericarditis in approximately 30 % of cases.

Siddiqui and Khan (2002) reported a case of isoniazid-induced lupus erythematosus presenting with cardiac tamponade. A 73-year-old man was treated with isoniazid for 8 months at a dose of 300 mg a day. The patient responded to the withdrawal of the isoniazid therapy and placement of a pericardial window. It was described drug-induced heart failure in advanced pulmonary tuberculosis (Daynes 1974), hyperuricaemia induced by ethambutol (Narang et al. 1983) and pyrazinamide (Solangi et al. 2004).

4.4 Important Drug Interactions

Many TB patients have concomitant illnesses. At the start of TB treatment, all patients should be asked about medicines they are currently taking. The most important interactions with anti-TB drugs are due to rifampicin. Rifampicin induces pathways that metabolize other drugs, thereby reducing the concentration and effect of those drugs. To maintain a therapeutic effect, dosages of the other drug(s) may need to be increased. When rifampicin is discontinued, its metabolism-inducing effect resolves within about 2 weeks, and dosages of the other drug(s) will need to be reduced (WHO 2014).

It was experimentally shown, that the antidiabetic drug metformin (MET) reduces the intracellular growth of Mtb. MET controls the growth of drug-resistant Mtb strains, increases production of mitochondrial reactive oxygen species, and facilitates phagosome-lysosome fusion. Moreover, in two separate human cohorts, MET treatment was associated with improved control of Mtb infection and decreased disease severity. Collectively, these data indicate that MET is a promising candidate host-adjunctive therapy for improving the effective treatment of TB (Singhal et al. 2014).

Worldwide anti-tuberculosis (TB) drug-induced liver disease (DILI) is an important cause of hepatotoxicity, and drug-induced acute liver failure (ALF). Antituberculosis drug-induced liver injury is a leading cause of DILI and drug-induced ALF in India (Saukkonen et al. 2006; Devarbhavi 2011). The liver has a central role in drug metabolism and detoxification, and is consequently vulnerable to injury. Anti-TB DILI occurs throughout treatment duration progressing to ALF in a quarter of patients. The overall mortality is 22.7 %, which is higher when accompanied by jaundice, ascites or encephalopathy. An anti-TB DILI model, incorporating bilirubin, INR, encephalopathy, serum creatinine and albumin predicted mortality with high level of the evidence.

The clinical spectrum includes asymptomatic elevation in liver tests to acute hepatitis and acute liver failure. TB DILI can occur across all age groups including children with significant morbidity and mortality. Although TB DILI develops more commonly in males, ALF is noted to be commoner in females with a worse prognosis. The combined affliction of HIV or chronic hepatitis B or C and tuberculosis poses multiple challenges including the greatly increased risks of DILI (Devarbhavi et al. 2013).

4.5 How to Improve Tolerance of the Therapy for Kidney Tuberculosis

Side effects (SE) of the anti-TB therapy in 117 patients with KTB were analyzed (Kul'chavenia and Kuznetsov 1998). KTB 3–4 stages was diagnosed in 79 (67.5 %), KTB 1–2 stages was – in 38 (32.5 %); 58 patients (49.6 %) had bilateral KTB. Patients were randomized on 2 groups. Ninety five patients were treated by intravenous administration of isoniazid and rifampicin plus intramuscular injection of streptomycin; also they took pyrazinamide per os (1st group). Twenty two patients received standard chemotherapy: isoniazid, pyrazinamide and rifampicin per os and intramuscular injection of streptomycin (2nd group).

Following complications of KTB were revealed: TB of ureter – in 17 patients (14.5 %), bladder TB – in 30 patients (25.6 %), chronic renal failure (CRF) – 24 patients (20.5 %).

Some co-morbidities were diagnosed: food allergy – in 34 patients (29.1 %), gastrointestinal tract diseases – in 18 patients (15.4 %), cordial system diseases – in 20 patients (17.1 %), pyelonephritis – in 12 patients (10.6 %), and chronic obstructive bronchitis – in 6 patients (5.1 %).

Among all 117 patients 48 (41.0 %) had SEs, mostly in the beginning of the therapy: in 1 month – 32 patients (66.7 %), and 6 patients (12.5 %) showed bad tolerance of anti-TB therapy in 2 months. In 1st group SEs were in 35 patients (36.8 %), and in 2nd group −13 patients (59.1 %) had SEs ($P<0.005$). More often SEs had women (62.5 %). Most toxic drugs were pyrazinamide (87.5 %), streptomycin (26.4 %). Isoniazid had bad tolerance in 18.2 %.

Bilateral KTB, CRF were factors of high risk of SEs development. But destructive forms as well as co-morbidity didn't show positive correlation with SEs.

Thus, anti-TB therapy for KTB is complicated by SEs in 41.0 %. Intravenous therapy has significantly better tolerance, than standard per os treatment. Most toxic drugs are pyrazinamide and streptomycin. Chance to have SE is higher in women with bilateral KTB, complicated by CRF.

References

Blair HA, Scott LJ (2015) Delamanid: a review of its use in patients with multidrug-resistant tuberculosis. Drugs 75(1):91–100. doi:10.1007/s40265-014-0331-4

Chepuri Nagaraj R, Kandi S, Sreenivas A, Oeltmann J, Satyanarayana S, Sachdeva KS, Motta Shamrao S (2013) A qualitative study to understand reasons for loss to follow-up during treatment for drug-resistant tuberculosis under programme conditions, Andhra Pradesh. Int J Tuberc Lung Dis 17(12 (suppl 2)):s 101

Chien J-Y, Lu MC, Chang YC, Ruiming H (2013) Hua-Lien Hospital, Department of Health, Executive Yuan, Hualien, Taiwan, outcome of rifabutin replacing intolerable rifampicin during anti-tuberculosis treatment. Int J Tuberc Lung Dis 17(12 (suppl 2)):s 156

Claasens M, Yang B, Dunbar R, Beyers N (2013) What determines initial loss to follow-up in tuberculosis patients at primary health care facilities in South Africa? Int J Tuberc Lung Dis 17(12 (suppl 2)):s 159

Daynes G (1974) Drug-induced heart failure in advanced pulmonary tuberculosis. S Afr Med J 48(57):2352–2353

de Souza AF, de Oliveira e Silva A, Baldi J, de Souza TN, Rizzo PM (1996) Hepatic functional changes induced by the combined use of isoniazid, pyrazinamide and rifampicin in the treatment of pulmonary tuberculosis. Arq Gastroenterol 33(4):194–200

Devarbhavi H (2011) Antituberculous drug-induced liver injury: current perspective. Trop Gastroenterol 32(3):167–174

Devarbhavi H, Singh R, Patil M, Sheth K, Adarsh CK, Balaraju G (2013) Outcome and determinants of mortality in 269 patients with combination anti-tuberculosis drug-induced liver injury. J Gastroenterol Hepatol 28(1):161–167. doi:10.1111/j.1440-1746.2012.07279.x

Dhingra VK, Rajpal S, Aggarwal N, Aggarwaln JK, Shadab K, Jain SK (2004) Adverse drug reactions observed during DOTS. J Commun Dis 36(4):251–259

Erokhin VV, Demikhova O, Bocharova IV, Severin ES, Barseghyan GG (2013) Preclinical trials of anti-tuberculosis drugs based on nanotechnology. Int J Tuberc Lung Dis 17(12 (suppl 2)):s 100

Grosset JH, Singer TG, Bishai WR (2012) New drugs for the treatment of tuberculosis: hope and reality. Int J Tuberc Lung Dis 16(8):1005–1014. doi:10.5588/ijtld.12.0277

Jindani A, Harherill M, Charalambous S, Mingofa S, Zizhou S, Van Dijk J, Shepherd J, Philips P (2013) Results of the Rifaquin study. Int J Tuberc Lung Dis 17(12 (suppl 2)):s 26

Kho VK, Chan PH (2012) Isolated tuberculous epididymitis presenting as a painless scrotal tumor. J Chin Med Assoc 75(6):292–295. doi:10.1016/j.jcma.2012.04.014.Epub2012May31

Kisonga R, Taksdal M, Kyariga N, Mleoh L (2013) The role of nutrition during MDR-TB patient's treatment. Int J Tuberc Lung Dis 17(12 (suppl 2)):s 19

Koizumi C, Suetomi T, Matsuoka T. et al (2014) Regional difference in cancer detection rate in prostate cancer screening by a local municipality in Japan. Prostate Int 2(1):19–25. doi:10.12954/PI.13035. [Epub 2014 Mar 30]

Kolpakova TA, Kolpakov MA, Bashkirova IV, Rachkovskaia LN, Burylin SI, Liubarskiĭ MS (2001) Effects of the enterosorbent SUMS-1 on isoniazid pharmacokinetics and lipid peroxidation in patients with pulmonary tuberculosis and drug-induced hepatic lesions. Probl Tuberk 3:34–36

Kombe R, Kapalata N (2013) Food prescription: experiences from food supplements in TB-HIV treatment in Temeke. Int J Tuberc Lung Dis 17(12 (suppl 2)):s 19

Kresyun V, Filyuk V, Antonenko P, Rogach K, Danilenko Y, Mozolevich G (2013) Level of isoniazid metabolites in tuberculosis patients depending on acetylation genotype. Int J Tuberc Lung Dis 17(12 (suppl 2)):s 158

Kul'chavenia EV, Kuznetsov PV (1998) Complications of polychemotherapy for renal tuberculosis. Probl Tuberk 1:28–30

Kulchavenya EV, Krasnov VA (2010) Selected issue of phthysiourology (Monograph). – Novosibirsk. "Nauka" ("Science") – ISBN 978-5-02-023313-3

Kwon OJ, Zhang L, Ittmann MM, Xin L (2014) Prostatic inflammation enhances basal-to-luminal differentiation and accelerates initiation of prostate cancer with a basal cell origin. Proc Natl Acad Sci U S A 111(5):E592–E600. doi:10.1073/pnas.1318157111. Epub 2013 Dec 23

Layer P, Engelhardm M (1986) Tuberculostatics-induced systemic lupus erythematosus. Dtsch Med Wochenschr 111(42):1603–1605

Liu X, Goldstein AS (2014) Inflammation promotes prostate differentiation. Proc Natl Acad Sci U S A 111(5):1666–1667. doi:10.1073/pnas.1323181111. Epub 2014 Jan 23

López Barón E, Gómez-Arbeláez D, Díaz-Pérez JA (2009) Primary prostatic tuberculosis. Case report and bibliographic review. Arch Esp Urol 62(4):309–313

Mirtskhulaya V, Lomtadze N, Kipiani M, Kavtaradze M, Salakaia A (2013) Factors associated with default from tuberculosis treatment in the country of Georgia: a case control study. Int J Tuberc Lung Dis 17(12 (suppl 2)):s 159

Mitchison DA (2003) Role of individual drugs in the chemotherapy of tuberculosis. Int J Tuberc Lung Dis 7(3):304

Mitchison D, Davies G (2012) The chemotherapy of tuberculosis: past, present and future. Int J Tuberc Lung Dis 16(6):724–732. doi:10.5588/ijtld.12.0083

Modongo C, Kesenogile B, Ncube R, Zetola N (2013) Effectiveness and toxicity of aminoglycoside use fro MDR-TB treatment: a matter of dead or deaf? Int J Tuberc Lung Dis 17(12 (suppl 2)):s 160

Mor Z, Cedar N, Leventhal A, Shuldiner J (2013) Are patients who recovered from tuberculosis still at risk of premature death? Results of a 10-year follow-up of all Israeli patients. Int J Tuberc Lung Dis 17(12 (suppl 2)):s 98

Narang RK, Agarwal MC, Raina AK, Singh SN, Bihari K, Sharma SN (1983) Hyperuricaemia induced by ethambutol. Br J Dis Chest 77(4):403–406

Olaru ID, von Groote-Bidlingmaier F, Heyckendorf J, Yew WW, Lange C, Chang KC (2014) Novel drugs against tuberculosis: a clinician's perspective. Eur Respir J, pii:erj01623-2014

Pereira RM, Tresoldi AT, Hessel G (2000) Isoniazid-induced hepatic failure. Report of a case. Arq Gastroenterol 37(1):72–75

Peto HM, Pratt RH, Harrington TA, LoBue PA, Armstrong LR (2009) Epidemiology of extrapulmonary tuberculosis in the United States, 1993–2006. Clin Infect Dis 49(9):1350–1357

Riva MA (2014) From milk to rifampicin and back again: history of failures and successes in the treatment for tuberculosis. J Antibiot Tokyo 67(9):661–665. doi:10.1038/ja.2014.108. Epub 2014 Aug 6

Saifullah B, El Zowalaty M, Arulselvan P, Fakurazi S, Webster T, Geilich M, Hussein MZ (2014) Antimycobacterial, antimicrobial, and biocompatibility properties of para-aminosalicylic acid with zinc layered hydroxide and Zn/Al layered double hydroxide nanocomposites. Drug Des Devel Ther 8:1029–1036. doi:10.2147/DDDT.S63753. Published online Jul 28, 2014

Sandhu JS (2008) Prostate cancer and chronic prostatitis. Curr Urol Rep 9(4):328–332

Saukkonen JJ, Cohn DL, Jasmer RM, Schenker S, Jereb JA, Nolan CM, Peloquin CA, Gordin FM, Nunes D, Strader DB, Bernardo J, Venkataramanan R, Sterling TR (2006) An official ATS statement: hepatotoxicity of antituberculosis therapy. Am J Respir Crit Care Med 174(8):935–952

Shean K, Upadhya D, van der Walt M (2013) Prevalence and severity of adverse reactions to clofazimine on the Western Cape province of South Africa. Int J Tuberc Lung Dis 17(12 (suppl 2)):s 262

Shutskaia EI, Priakhina VN, Kolpakova TA, Kurilovich GM (1991) Drug-induced nephropathy in patients with tuberculosis of the lungs. Probl Tuberk 4:48–49

Siddiqui MA, Khan IA (2002) Isoniazid-induced lupus erythematosus presenting with cardiac tamponade. Am J Ther 9(2):163–165

Silberstein T, Silberstein E, Saphier O (2013) Lycopene and tomatoes–their effect on prevention of prostatic cancer. Harefuah 152(8):461–463, 499

Simons BW, Durham NM, Bruno TC et al (2015) A human prostatic bacterial isolate alters the prostatic microenvironment and accelerates prostate cancer progression. J Pathol 235(3): 478–489. doi: 10.1002/path.4472

Singhal A, Jie L, Kumar P, Hong GS, Leow MK, Paleja B, Tsenova L, Kurepina N, Chen J, Zolezzi F, Kreiswirth B, Poidinger M, Chee C, Kaplan G, Wang YT, De Libero G (2014) Metformin as adjunct antituberculosis therapy. Sci Transl Med 6(263):263ra159. doi:10.1126/scitranslmed.3009885

Solangi GA, Zuberi BF, Shaikh S, Shaikh WM (2004) Pyrazinamide induced hyperuricemia in patients taking anti-tuberculous therapy. J Coll Physicians Surg Pak 14(3):136–138

Svensson EM, Murray S, Karlsson MO, Dooley KE (2014) Rifampicin and rifapentine significantly reduce concentrations of bedaquiline, a new anti-TB drug. J Antimicrob Chemother. pii:dku504

Tang S, Hao X, Yao L, Liu Y, Sun H, Gu J (2013a) Clofazimine for the treatment of multidrug-resistant tuberculosis: a multicenter, randomized controlled study. Int J Tuberc Lung Dis 17(12 (suppl 2)):s 155

Tang S, Yao L, Hao X, Liu Y, Sun H, Gu J (2013b) Linezolid for the treatment of extensively drug-resistant tuberculosis: a multicenter, randomized controlled study. Int J Tuberc Lung Dis 17(12 (suppl 2)):s 160

Thee S, Garcia-Prats A, Draper HR, McIlleron H, Meredith S, Wiesner L, Hesseling A, Schaaf HS (2013) Pharmacokinetics of ofloxacin and levofloxacin in children with multi-drug resistant tuberculosis. Int J Tuberc Lung Dis 17(12 (suppl 2)):s 255

van der Werf MJ, Langendam MW, Huitric E (2013) Role of adherence to tuberculosis treatment guidelines to prevent the development of drug resistance. Int J Tuberc Lung Dis 17(12 (suppl 2)):s 41

Vilaplana C, Cardona PJ (2013) Could the common anti-inflammatories be the new coadjuvant treatment against tuberculosis? Int J Tuberc Lung Dis 17(12 (suppl 2)):s 157

Vishnevskyi BI, Steklova LN (2008) Frequency and structure of drug resistance of M. tuberculosis in different localizations of the disease. Probl tuberculeza i bolezn legkih 12:5–8

WHO (1991) WHO model prescribing information: drugs used in mycobacterial diseases. WHO, Geneva

WHO (2013) WHO model list of essential medicines. World Health Organization. http://apps.who.int/iris/bitstream/10665/93142/1/EML_18_eng.pdf?ua=1

WHO (2013) Countdown to 2015; Global Tuberculosis Report 2013, Supplement 2013. WHO/HTM/TB/2013.13. WHO, Geneva

WHO Fact sheet N°104, Reviewed March 2014, available on http://www.who.int/mediacentre/factsheets/fs104/en/

Zierski M, Bek E (1980) Side effects of various combinations of rifampin and isoniazid with ethambutol or streptomycin and pyrazinamide in short-term chemotherapy of newly-detected pulmonary tuberculosis. Pneumonol Pol 48(7):469–479

Chapter 5
Regimens of the Chemotherapy for Urogenital Tuberculosis

Abstract Treatment of TB requires administration of several drugs for at least 6–12 months, and in special cases – to 18–24 months leading to high costs, side-effects and the emergence of drug-resistant strains associated with patient non-compliance.

Regimen of the chemotherapy (ChT) for UGTB strongly depends on the form of the disease; nevertheless there are some general principles: (1) Choice optimal drugs; and (2) Choice an optimal administration of the drugs. Optimal anti-TB drugs for UGTB are: isoniazid (intravenous or intramuscular injection), rifampicin (intrevenously or in micro-enema), pyrazinamide per os, fluoroquinolones: levofloxacin / ofloxacin (intravenously or per os), PAS (intravenously) (especially for bladder TB and prostate TB), amycacin i.m. (especially in co-morbidity with non-specific pyelonephritis), cycloserin per os (especially in co-morbidity with non-specific pyelonephritis) amoxicillin/clavulanate, meropenem, imipenem, clarithromycin.

Again, the main principles of anti-TB chemotherapy are: continuity, controllability, succession of the treatment. The patient has to take minimum four anti-TB drugs simultaneously during a minimum of 6 months, depending on the form of UGTB.

Keywords Urogenital tuberculosis • Therapy • Anti-TB drugs • Regimens • Intravenous chemotherapy • Outcome

5.1 Introduction

Effective chemotherapy rapidly reduced population of viable bacilli and consequently reduces the risk of transmission – so, again, TB as whole and UGTB particularly are fully cured – but there are some special condition for this, and told about it earlier. No known chemotherapeutic agent possesses each of these properties to a degree that renders it self-sufficient for the recovery. At least three drugs should be administered concomitantly for the first 2 months, in particular to prevent the emergence of resistance, and in all cases treatment must be continued with at least two drugs for several months longer before there can be reasonable assurance of cure (WHO 2014).

E. Kulchavenya, *Current Therapy and Surgery for Urogenital Tuberculosis*,
DOI 10.1007/978-3-319-28290-9_5

5.2 Principles of the Chemotherapy for UGTB

Treatment of TB requires administration of several drugs for at least 6–12 months, and in special cases – to 18–24 months leading to high costs, side-effects and the emergence of drug-resistant strains associated with patient non-compliance.

The management of the patients with TB is challenging in several respects:

1. Mtb are vulnerable to anti-TB drugs only when they are metabolically active and replicating.
2. Small subpopulation of Mtb always remains semidormant indefinitely long time. They become transiently active – and thus vulnerable to anti-TB drugs – for very short period of time, and we have to do all our best to provide enough concentration of bactericidal agents this time exactly. Mtb is very capricious, and if the conditions are poor, Mtb will not replicate.
3. Drug-resistant mutant can exist even in population of bacilli never previously exposed to antibiotic – so called "previous", or "wild" resistance.

We have a number of very strong anti-TB drugs – but results are often poor. Why? Particularly, because of peculiarities of TB infection determine a special approach to the chemotherapy of urogenital tuberculosis.

First, we cannot treat "UGTB" – we have to define special therapy for each form of UGTB, alike for urinary tract infections (UTI), which combine diseases from urethritis and cystitis till urosepsis – and each form should be treated differently.

Second, the beginning of the ChT immediately compels Mtb to reduce its replication, and slow- or non-replicating bacteria in hypoxic granulomas are phenotypically tolerant towards antibiotics (Raffetseder et al. 2014). Even small doses of anti-TB drugs, including amicacin and fluoroquinolones, which are widely used in general urology, make living conditions unpleasant for Mtb and its transfers into dormant form – insensitive to antimycobacterials. It is one more reason for the long time anti-TB treatment – we try to catch the moment of the replication of mycobacteria, when they are sensible to the action of anti-TB drugs. The problem is – we cannot predict this moment. It may be in one day, in one week, in one month and even in one year.

There are two exits from this problem:

- We maintain high dose concentration of anti-TB drug for a long time continuously –whenever Mtb wake up from dormancy – anti-TB drugs kill its;
- We manage therapy in intermittent regimen. In days of administration of anti-TB drugs active Mtb will be killed, dormant Mtb remain persistent. During 2–3 days without therapy (cleaning period) some of dormant Mtb become active – because of inhibiting effect of anti-TB drugs stopped – and new dose of anti-TB drug will kill new portion of Mtb. Basis of the intermittent anti-TB therapy for pulmonary TB patients and evidence of its efficiency were made in Novosibirsk Research TB Institute (Russia) in 70–80-th last century under supervision of prof. Igor Ursov (1991).

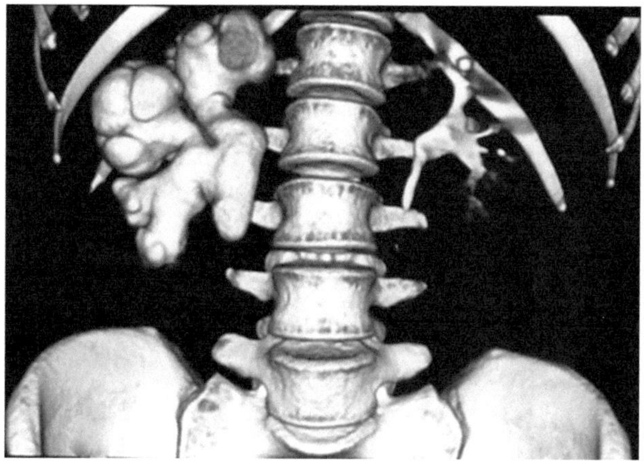

Fig. 5.1 Multi-slice tomogram of UGTB patient (KTB-2 on the right, complicated by TB of ureter). Post-tuberculous pyelonephritis, post-tuberculous stricture of the right ureter, hydronephrosis on the right

Third, drugs poor penetrate fibrous wall of a cavern and its concentration in caseous mass is low, insufficient for destroying of Mtb. To overcome this obstacle we can via address delivery of anti-TB drugs.

And finally, healing of TB is occurs via forming fibrosis. It is a good outcome for pulmonary TB – but not for UGTB, where we receive "desirable fibrosis in undesirable place". Sequels of UGTB, such as stricture of ureter or urethra, shrinkage of bladder etc. may be more serious than proper TB inflammation. Inappropriate management of UGTB patient results in loss of organ, even if TB is cured. The example of post-tuberculous hydronephrosis due to post-tuberculosis stricture of ureter is shown on Fig. 5.1.

Regimen of the ChT for UGTB strongly depends on the form of the disease; nevertheless there are two very important points: (1) Choice of optimal drugs; and (2) Choice of optimal administration of the drugs.

5.3 How to Choose the Optimal Anti-TB Drugs

Not all anti-TB drugs are suitable for all forms of UGTB. Standard scheme recommended by WHO (isoniazid + rifampicin + pyrazinamide + streptomycin/ethambutol) is good for simple non-complicated cases only. For example, kidney TB 1 stage, when there are some granulomas without destruction of parenchyma. Streptomycin is not optimal for complicated forms of UGTB, when urinary tract is involved, as it lead to redundant fibrosis and forming of strictures. Ethambutol is not optimal in kidney TB 2–4 stages, when hematuria is common symptom, as it provokes hematuria. As well ethambutol poor penetrates prostatic tissue and cannot provide sufficient concentration in the site of inflammation in patients with prostate TB.

Thus, streptomycin and kanamycin are not recommended for UGTB; among fluoroquinolones ofloxacin or levofloxacin only are suitable for UGTB therapy.

Moxifloxacin and sparfloxacin are respiratory fluoroquinolones, so they are good for PTB, but not optimal for UGTB.

PAS is highly recommended for UGTB with involvement of pelvic organs, amoxicillin/clavulonat should be prescribed together with meropenem or imipenem, as they potentiate anti-TB effect. Cycloserin is highly recommended, if the patient has comorbidity of UGTB and non-specific UTI. Patient with comorbidity of UGTB and HIV and receiving anti-retrovirus therapy should be treated with rifabutin instead of rifampicin. Rifampicin and streptomycin are contraindicated for patients after organ transplantation. Amikacin as well as streptomycin and kanamycin are contraindicated for UTTB patients.

Optimal anti-TB drugs for UGTB are:

- Isoniazid (intravenous or intramuscular injection)
- Rifampicin (intrevenously or per rectum)
- Pyrazinamide per os
- Fluoroquinolones: levofloxacin / ofloxacin (intravenously or per os)
- PAS (intravenously or per os) (especially for BTB and PTB)
- Amycacin i.m. (especially in co-morbidity with non-specific pyelonephritis)
- Cycloserin per os (especially in co-morbidity with non-specific pyelonephritis) amoxicillin/clavulanate
- meropenem
- imipenem
- clarithromycin.

Of course, we can use any other anti-TB drug – but with precaution. There is no any data on using new anti-TB drugs bedaquilin and perhlozon in UGTB patients, so we cannot recommend its yet.

5.4 How to Choose the Optimal Administration of Anti-TB Drugs

Simplest and cheapest way of administration of anti-TB drugs is intake per os. It is suitable when you have many patients and a few personnel and finances. But it is not optimal. UGTB is local form of TB, and address delivery of drugs is preferable. It may be achieved by using liposomal forms, by lymphotropic, including rectal, or intravenous administration.

Again, the main principles of anti-TB chemotherapy are: continuity, controllability, succession of the treatment. The patient has to take at least four anti-TB drugs simultaneously during at least 2 months (intensive phase) followed by phase continuation for at least 6 months with at least two anti-TB drugs, depending on the form of UGTB. Of course compliance is low and some patients try to avoid receiving these drugs. When they receive pills – nurse cannot be exact sure they swallow its. When she introduce drugs intramuscular, intravenous, or rectal – she fully control the therapy. Neglecting of these principles leads to development of drug-resistance of Mtb and relapse of TB.

Table 5.1 Standard schemes of a chemotherapy for UGTB

Regime	Phase	
	Intensive	Continuation
I	2 H R Z E / Am	4 H R / 6 H_3 R_3
II	1 H Z R Ofl/Lef Cs/Am	5 H Z R / 6 H_3 R_3 E_3
	+2 H Z R Cs/Am	
III	2 H Z R Ofl/Lef Cs/PAS	4 H Z R / 5 H_3 R_3 E_3
	+2 H Z R Cs/PAS	
IV	4 Cap Z Ofl/Lef Cs /PAS /Pt(Et) +	6 E Z PAS/ Pt(Et)
	2 Cap Z Cs /PAS /Pt(Et)	
V	Accordingly to sensitivity of Mtb	Not less than 4 drugs
	Not less than 5 drugs	E Pt Ofl/Lef Rb Cs PAS[Amx Imp Clr Mp]
	6–8 Cap Z Ofl/Lef Cs /PAS /Pt(Et)/ E / Rb/ /Cs	Length not less than 18 mo.
	[Amx Imp Clr Mp]	

5.5 Etiotropic Therapy for UGTB

The etiotropic therapy for UGTB differs from the therapy of PTB. Depending on the form of UGTB 5 regimes of chemotherapy are defined:

Regime I is applied in new-revealed treatment-naive patients with drug-susceptible (or if there was no growth of Mtb) non-complicated KTB 1–2 stages, isolated TB epididymitis, patients who were diagnosed by histology after organ-removed surgery performed in general urology, if there is no other TB focus.

Regime II is applied in new-revealed treatment-naive patients with drug-susceptible (or if there was no growth of Mtb) non-complicated KTB 3–4 stages.

Regime III is applied in new-revealed treatment-naive patients with drug-susceptible (or if there was no growth of Mtb) KTB 4 stage, KTB any stage complicated by UTTB, prostate TB, gUGTB.

Regime IV is applied in patients with relapse of UGTB, with high risk of MDR, independent on stage and form.

Regime V is applied in patients with MDR-UGTB, independent on the stage and form.

Every regime includes the phase of intensive therapy followed by the continuation phase (see Table 5.1).

5.5.1 Doses of Anti-TB Drugs

WHO recommends fixed dose combination of anti-TB drugs and proposes standardized daily dosage for body weight, but these doses are, on the opinion of many National guidelines, suboptimal. So, in Russian Federation isoniazid is used in

Table 5.2 Recommended daily dosage of antituberculous drugs for adults (mg)

The drug	Patient's weight		
	33–50 kg	51–70 kg	More than 70 kg max
Isoniazid	300	300–600	600
Rifampicin	450	450–600	600
Pyrazinamide	1000–1500	1500–2000	2500
Amikacin	500–750	1000	1000
Ethambutol	800–1200	1200–1600	1600–2000
Levofloxacin	500	500–750	750–1000
Ofloxacin	400–800	800	800–1000
Protionamid/etionamid	500	750	750–1000
Capreomycin	500–750	750–1000	1000
PAS	3000–5000	5000–8000	8000–12,000
Cycloserin	500	500–750	750–1000

twofold dose; National TB Program of Thailand accepted higher doze pyrazinamide (30 mg/kg/day). Prospective study has shown that this dose of pyrazinamide didn't lead to the increasing of the frequency of side effects, but incidence rate of pyrazinamide-induced hepatotoxicity was highest with dosing >30–40 mg/kg/day (Onpum and Pungraddami 2013).

The dosage depends on the weight; recommended ones are given in the Table 5.2.

Anti-TB drugs may be prescribed *per os*, but parenteral administration (optimal intravenous infusion) is preferable, as it provides better control and minimizes side effects.

5.5.2 *Intravenous Administration*

We cannot avoid prescription of at least four drugs simultaneously, but we have to optimize their choice and optimize a method of administration. We can get over limits of the chemotherapy by intravenous treatment.

Intravenous drop-by-drop (stream) administration of anti-TB drugs resulted in the therapy intensification allowing accelerating the sputum/urine/ejaculate conversion and cavities closure in PTB (caverns in kidneys and in prostate remain forever; there is now a method to closure them by medications). The method of intravenous infusion is based on the possibility to create very high concentration of the drugs in blood plasma omitting liver as the principal organ of the drugs inactivation.

During the intravenous infusion the concentration of the drugs in tissue, including kidney and prostate parenchyma, exceeds considerably the bacteriostatic level of the oral and even intramuscular administration. Although high concentration of the drugs in the blood is not too long, it helps to increase their enhanced diffusion to the zone of TB inflammation. This method allows creating sufficient bacteriostatic and even bactericide concentration even in the caseous foci that are difficult for the drug access.

Advantages of Intravenous Anti-TB Therapy
Advantages of intravenous anti-TB therapy are:

- full dose of the drugs gets blood plasma omitting liver;
- it is possible to create the required concentration of the ant-TB drugs in the organs for definite time depending on the drugs infusion rate;
- it avoids negative influence on gastrointestinal tract, that is especially important for the patients with concomitant gastrointestinal tract diseases, as they often tolerate badly or do not tolerate the oral administration of the antibiotics;
- the duration of hospital treatment is reducing;
- the drug resistance to Mtb, some SE are less frequent;
- best control of the therapy allows excluding the irregular taking of the drugs and defaults.

Anti-TB Drugs Suitable for Intravenous Administration
There are the following anti-TB drugs suitable for intravenous administration:

- isoniazid,
- rifampicin (as rifamycin SV sodium),
- ethambutol,
- PAS (para-aminosalicylic acid),
- soluble salt of ethionamide,
- fluoroquinolones (ofloxacin, levofloxacin, moxifloxacin),
- linezolid.

Improved drug delivery systems are probably the best solution for treating TB as they can improve drug bioavailability for longer time periods and release the drug in a sustained local manner to avoid toxicity.

Liposomal Forms of Anti-TB Drugs
Treatment of tuberculosis remains challenging, with lengthy treatment durations and complex drug regimens that are toxic and difficult to administer. Similar to the vast majority of antibiotics, drugs for *Mycobacterium tuberculosis* are directed against microbial targets. Although more effective drugs that target the bacterium may lead to faster cure of patients, it is possible that a biological limit will be reached that can be overcome only by adopting a fundamentally new treatment approach. Greco et al. (2012) have generated unique asymmetric liposomes with phosphatidylserine (PS) distributed at the outer membrane surface to resemble apoptotic bodies and phosphatidic acid (PA) at the inner layer as a strategy to enhance innate antimycobacterial activity in phagocytes while limiting the inflammatory response. TB regimens might be improved by including agents that target host pathways. Recent work on host-pathogen interactions, host immunity, and host-directed interventions suggests that supplementing anti-TB therapy with host modulators may lead to shorter treatment times, a reduction in lung damage caused by the disease, and a lower risk of relapse or reinfection (Hawn et al. 2013).

The combination of liposomes with polymeric scaffolds could revolutionize the current state of drug delivery technology. Over the past few decades, liposomes have received widespread attention as a carrier system for therapeutically active compounds, due to their unique characteristics such as capability to incorporate hydrophilic and hydrophobic drugs, good biocompatibility, low toxicity, lack of immune system activation, and targeted delivery of bioactive compounds to the site of action (Mufamadi et al. 2011).

Another results showed that the reduction of the level of infection was more dependent on the administered dose than on the number of doses administered per week. The incorporation of rifabutin into liposomes seems to be a very promising therapeutic system for the treatment or prophylaxis of infectious diseases. The intravenous administration of liposomal rifabutin to mice infected with*M. avium* resulted in a greater reductions in the level of infection compared to the administration of the RFB in the free form either before or after the establishment of infection (Gaspar et al. 2000).

Efficacy of liposome-encapsulated amikacin and free amikacin against Mycobacterium avium complex was evaluated in the beige mouse acute infection model. Compared with free amikacin, encapsulated amikacin significantly reduced viable cell counts in the liver and spleen. Liposome encapsulation of an active agent appears to be a promising therapeutic approach to M. avium complex infection (Cynamon et al. 1989).

The therapeutic efficacy of liposomal clofazimine (L-CLF) was studied by Adams et al. (1999) in mice infected with *Mycobacterium tuberculosis* Erdman. Authors have found a highly effective therapeutic response of L-CLF alone against *M. tuberculosis* infection in acute, established, and chronic murine models; the absence of recurrence of *M. tuberculosis* growth suggested a bactericidal effect of L-CLF in the liver and spleen. They therefore believe that L-CLF can be used as an effective therapeutic agent for the treatment of *M. tuberculosis* infections.

The efficacies of isoniazid and rifampin encapsulated in lung-specific stealth liposomes were evaluated by injecting liposomal drugs and free drugs into tuberculous mice twice a week for 6 weeks. Liposome-encapsulated drugs at and below therapeutic concentrations were more effective than free drugs against tuberculosis. Furthermore, liposomal drugs had marginal hepatotoxicities as determined from the levels of total bilirubin and hepatic enzymes in serum. The elimination of Mtb from the liver and spleen was also higher with liposomal drugs than with free drugs. The encapsulation of anti-TB drugs in lung-specific stealth liposomes seems to be a promising therapeutic approach for the chemotherapy of TB (Deol et al. 1997).

5.6 Etiotropic Therapy for Prostate Tuberculosis

Prostate tuberculosis (PTB) is difficult for early diagnostic as far as both clinical features and laboratory findings (excluding M. tuberculosis) are non-specific. PTB seems to be a rare disease. Nevertheless, 70 % of men died from tuberculosis of all localizations had prostate tuberculosis mostly overlooked during life time (Kamyshan 2003). For example in Russia it is more than 10,000 men annually – and prostate tuberculosis is a sexually transmitted disease and one of the main reasons for infertility – both male and female (Kulchavenya and Krasnov 2010). The results of the therapy closely depends on in-time diagnostic – if patient is revealed in stage of cavern, he will never be fully cured. Standard chemotherapy for PTB is insufficiently effective: only 22.8 % of patients were cured with isoniazid, rifampicin, pyrazinamid and streptomycin, and in 77.2 % disease became chronic (Kulchavenya and Khomyakov 2006).

Efficiency of optimized scheme for the therapy of BTB was estimated in 53 patients in the age of 24–69 years (Kulchavenya et al. 2014). All patients were randomized on two groups. First group (25 patients) was treated with a standard scheme of chemotherapy: isoniazid in dose 10 mg/kg + pyrazinamid in dose 25 mg/kg + streptomycin 1.0 + rifampicin in dose 10 mg/kg in intensive phase (2 months), and isoniazid and rifampicin in phase continuation. Second group (28 PTB patients) alongside with standard chemotherapy received ofloxacin in dose 10 mg/kg during intensive phase. The phase continuation was in both groups identical, with rifampicin and isoniazid for 6 months.

Optimization of the standard therapy by additional administration of ofloxacin improved results of the treatment on 33.8 %: patients in optimized group got good results in 77.8 %, but in standard one – in 44.0 %.

The therapy of prostatitis any etiology – both non-specific and tuberculous is very difficult as a few antibacterial agents are able to distribute to the prostatic tissue and achieve sufficient concentrations at the site of infection. These agents include fluoroquinolones, macrolides, tetracyclines and trimethoprim (Magri et al. 2013). Standard anti-TB drugs, excluding rifampicin, have sub-optimal concentration in prostate tissue (Kulchavenya and Krasnov 2010), but ofloxacin has wide antibacterial activity, including bactericidal effect on Mtb, so it is optimal drug for patients with PTB. Our results confirmed superiority of optimized polychemotherapy for patients with prostate TB in comparison with standard one.

The problem of early diagnosis is acute since 54.7 % of patients were revealed with caverns, when full, complete convalescence is impossible, and on contrary, relapse and chronic course are probable. For in-time diagnosis we have to follow main principals: careful study epidemic history of the patient, 3-glass test (Kulchavenya et al. 2012), performed before digital rectal examination, investigation of expressed prostatic fluid and ejaculate as well as prostate biopsies on M. tuberculosis by PCR.

Lee et al. (2001) estimated 18 patients (mean age 66.7 ± 10.2 years) with prostate tuberculosis to characterize the clinical features and to evaluate the short and long-term results of antituberculous chemotherapy. The median pretreatment PSA level was 2.7 ng/mL (range 0.3–31). Eight patients (44.4 %) received a triple-drug regimen of rifampin, ethambutol, and isoniazid for more than 6 months. The mean duration of chemotherapy was 7.6 months (range 6–12). Of the eight patients, three underwent chemotherapy longer because of concurrent tuberculosis of other organs. Follow-up studies included digital rectal examination, total PSA determination, and transrectal prostate biopsy. Ten patients were eligible for regular follow-up. The average number of follow-up transrectal prostate biopsies was 2.4 (range 2–3). The follow-up histologic findings showed nodular hyperplasia in seven patients and chronic inflammatory cell infiltration in three patients. No acid-fast bacillus was found in any follow-up specimen (Lee et al. 2001).

5.7 Can We Predict the Outcome of the Therapy?

Unfortunately, in spite of poly-components anti-TB chemotherapy, many patients die of TB. Drain et al. (2013) offered a rapid urine lipoarabinomannan test during TB treatment as a prognostic marker for mortality among TB patients. They have that a strongly positive rapid urine lipoarabinomannan test after 2 months of TB therapy independently predicts mortality among TB patients. HIV and TB co-infected patients who remain positive urine lipoarabinomannan test after 2 months of TB therapy may warrant closer follow-up visits or more intensive medical care.

This method is not yet approved and is not evident in good study, although it is promised. But can we really predict the outcome of the chemotherapy for TB? Can we be sure that standard therapy will be equally effective in all treated patients? I'm afraid, not at all, and there are many reasons for such pessimism. As we told above, there are three types of the metabolism of isoniazid. So patients with fast metabolism and patient with slow metabolism who took the same dose 0,6 isoniazid per os, actually received in first case about 0,3 and in second – about 0,9. Patient with fast metabolism will have low efficiency and good tolerance, and patient with slow metabolism will have good efficiency and high level of toxicity. And the dose was the same!

Marked interindividual variability was observed in the plasma concentrations of isoniazid, rifampicin and pyrazinamide at two hours after drug administration (Ruesen et al. 2014). Nevertheless the authors have no found the association between drug concentration and 8 weeks culture conversion, although low pyrazinamide concentration was associated with a less favourable bacteriological response.

Treatment cure and success rates were significantly higher among female TB patients compared to male patients. Male TB patients were more likely to die and failure from TB (Qader et al. 2013).

5.8 Pathogenetic Therapy

Some pathogenetic medications are used as additional treatment: tocopferol, canephron; trospium chloride for bladder TB 3 stage, afala and prostanorm for prostate TB etc (Kulchavenya 2014).

5.8.1 *Vitamin D in the Complex Anti-TB Therapy*

TB patients are commonly vitamin D deficient which may impact immunity. Vitamin D enhances host protective immune responses to Mtb by suppressing interferon-gamma and reducing disease – associated inflammation. Double blind randomized, controlled study in adult TB patients was carried out in Tbilisi. Vitamin D in the dose 1400000 IU per day was safe but didn't improve TB clearance in the overall cohort of the patients. However, patients with MDR-TB, who received vitamin D, demonstrated a shorter time to culture conversion (Tukvadze et al. 2015). On contrary, Hasan et al. (2013) presented evidence of superiority 600000 IU of vitamin D on placebo. Supplementation with 600,000 IU of vitamin D accelerated clinical, radiographic improvement in all TB patients and increased host immune activation in patients with baseline "deficient" sedum vitamin D levels. It should be noted, that this study was poorer designed, than one of Tukvadze et al. (2013), which looks more convincing.

While Canada has a lower incidence of TB, it adopt migrants from TB-endemic countries, who account for 66 % of all nation's cases (Boffa et al. 2013). For example, in Calgary extra-pulmonary tuberculosis (EPTB) occurs in 90 % among of foreign-born. The authors analyzed histories of 162 patients, and found, that only 13 % had sufficient vitamin D level, but 76 % had moderate, and 10 % had severely deficient vitamin D level. Among cases, 55 % had EPTB. Those with severe vitamin D deficiency had 3.14 greater odds of developing EPTB compared with moderate or sufficient vitamin D level (Boffa et al. 2013).

References

Adams LB, Sinha I, Franzblau SG, Krahenbuhl JL, Mehta RT (1999) Effective treatment of acute and chronic murine tuberculosis with liposome-encapsulated clofazimine. Antimicrob Agents Chemother 43(7):1638–1643

Boffa J, Moules N, Mayan M, Cowie RL (2013) More than just great quotes: an introduction to the Canadian Tri-Council's qualitative requirements. Can J Infect Dis Medicrobiol 24(2):103–8

Cynamon MH, Swenson CE, Palmer GS, Ginsberg RS (1989) Liposome-encapsulated-amikacin therapy of Mycobacterium avium complex infection in beige mice. Antimicrob Agents Chemother 33(8):1179–1183

Deol P, Khuller GK, Joshi K (1997) Therapeutic efficacies of isoniazid and rifampin encapsulated in lung-specific stealth liposomes against Mycobacterium tuberculosis infection induced in mice. Antimicrob Agents Chemother 41(6):1211–1214

Drain PK, Losina E, Parker G, Giddy J, Ross D, Katz JN, Coleman SM, Bogart LM, Freedberg KA, Walensky RP, Bassett IV (2013) Risk factors for late-stage HIV disease presentation at initial HIV diagnosis in Durban, South Africa. PLoS One 8(1), e55305. doi:10.1371/journal.pone.0055305, Epub 2013 Jan 28

Gaspar MM, Neves S, Portaels F, Pedrosa J, Silva MT, Cruz MEM (2000) Therapeutic efficacy of liposomal rifabutin in a *Mycobacterium avium* model of infection. Antimicrob Agents Chemother 44(9):2424–2430

Greco E, Quintiliani G, Santucci MB, Serafino A, Ciccaglione AR et al (2012) Janus-faced liposomes enhance antimicrobial innate immune response in Mycobacterium tuberculosis infection. Proc Natl Acad Sci U S A 109(21):E1360–E1368. doi:10.1073/pnas.1200484109. Published online Apr 25, 2012

Hasan Z, Rao N, Salahuddin N, Ali F, Aqeel M (2013) Vitamin D accelerates clinical recovery from tuberculosis: results of the SUCCINCT Study. Int J TB Lung Dis 17(12 (suppl 2)):s 261

Hawn TR, Matheson AI, Maley SN, Vandal O (2013) Host-directed therapeutics for tuberculosis: can we harness the host? Microbiol Mol Biol Rev 77(4):608–627. doi:10.1128/MMBR.00032-13

Htike W, Islam MA, Hasan MT, Ferdous S, Rifat M. Htike W, Islam MA, Hasan MT, Ferdous S, Rifat M (2013) Factors associated with treatment delay amongtuberculosis patients referred from a tertiary hospital in Dhaka City: a cross-sectional study. Public Health Action 3(4):317–22. doi:10.5588/pha.13.0067

Kamyshan IS (2003) Guideline on tuberculosis of urogenital organs. Kiev, 212

Kulchavenya E (2014) Urogenital tuberculosis: epidemiology, diagnosis, therapy. Springer, Cham/Heidelberg/New York/Dordrecht/London, 137pp. ISBN 978-2-319-04836-9. doi:10.1007/978-3-319-04837-6

Kulchavenya E, Khomyakov V (2006) Male genital tuberculosis in Siberians. World J Urol 24(1):74–78. Epub 2006 Jan 21

Kulchavenya EV, Krasnov VA (2010) Selected issue of phthysiourology (Monograph). – Novosibirsk, "Nauka" ("Science") – ISBN 978-5-02-023313-3

Kulchavenya E, Azizoff A, Brizhatyuk E, Khomyakov V, Kholtobin D, Breusoff A, Naber KG (2012) Improved diagnostics of chronic inflammatory prostatitis. Minerva Urol Nefrol 64:273–278

Kulchavenya E, Brizhatyuk E, Khomyakov V (2014) Diagnosis and therapy for prostate tuberculosis. Ther Adv Urol 6(4):129–134. doi:10.1177/1756287214529005

Lee Y, Huang W, Huang J, Wang J, Yu C, Jiaan B, Huang J (2001) Efficacy of chemotherapy for prostatic tuberculosis-a clinical and histologic follow-up study. Urology 57(5):872–877

Magri V, Wagenlehner FM, Marras E, van Till JW, Houbiers J, Panagopoulos P, Petrikkos GL, Perletti G (2013) Influence of infection on the distribution patterns of NIH-Chronic prostatitis symptom index scores in patients with chronic prostatitis/chronic pelvic pain syndrome (CP/CPPS). Exp Ther Med 6(2):503–508. Epub 2013 Jun 21

Mufamadi MS, Pillay V, Choonara YE, Du Toit LC, Modi G, Naidoo D, Ndesendo VMK (2011) A review on composite liposomal technologies for specialized drug delivery. J Drug Deliv 2011:939851. doi:10.1155/2011/939851. Published online Feb 8, 2011

Onpum A, Pungraddami P (2013) Pyrazinamide-induced hepatotoxicity: caution when using recommended daily dosage for body weight bands. Int J TB Lung Dis 17(12 (suppl 2)):s158

Qader GQ, Rashidi M, Mahmoodi M, Seddiq M, Hamim A, Momand A, Suarez PG, Enayatullah E (2013) Exploring tuberculosis treatment outcome distribution by gender in Afghanistan, 2009–2011. Int J TB Lung Dis 17(12 (suppl 2)):S 329

Raffetseder J, Pienaar E, Blomgran R, Eklund D, Patcha Brodin V, Andersson H, Welin A, Lerm M (2014 Nov 11) Replication rates of Mycobacterium tuberculosis in human macrophages do not correlate with mycobacterial antibiotic susceptibility. PLoS One 9(11), e112426. doi:10.1371/journal.pone.0112426.eCollection2014

Ruesen C, van Gageldonk-Lafeber AB, de Vries G, Erkens CG, van Rest J, Korthals Altes H, de Neeling H, Kamst M, van Soolingen D (2014) Extent and origin of resistance to antituberculosis drugs in the Netherlands, 1993 to 2011. Euro Surveill 19(11). pii: 20738

Tukvadze N, Sanikidze E, Kipiani M, Hebbar G, Easley KA, Shenvi N, Kempker RR, Frediani JK, Mirtskhulava V, Alvarez JA, Lomtadze N, Vashakidze L, Hao L, Del Rio C, Tangpricha V, Blumberg HM, Ziegler TR (2015) High-dose vitamin D3 in adults with pulmonary tuberculosis: a double-blind randomized controlled trial. Am J Clin Nutr 102(5):1059–69. doi:10.3945/ajcn.115.113886, Epub 2015 Sep 23

Ursov IG (1991) Can we confirm that tuberculosis has been cured? Probl Tuberk 5(5):18–20. Russian

WHO Fact sheet N°104, Reviewed March 2014, available on http://www.who.int/mediacentre/factsheets/fs104/en/

Chapter 6
Surgery for UGTB

Abstract UGTB is an often contracted, but mostly overlooked, disease. The main reasons for late diagnosis are lack of alertness on UGTB in urologists and general practitioners relative to patients with UTI, kidney anomalies, renal cysts etc.; non-specific variable clinical features, decreasing positive cultures of MBT due to non-optimal empiric therapy for UTI with prescribing of fluoroquinolones and amicacin.

Standard chemotherapy is effective only for early diagnosed forms of UGTB, in complicated form modified schemes with five anti-TB drugs in combination with pathogenetic therapy is indicated. Destructive forms of kidney and male genital TB cannot be cured by chemotherapy, surgery is necessary. Although chemotherapy is the mainstay of treatment, ablative surgery as a first-line management may be unavoidable for sepsis or abscesses. In cases with hydronephrosis and progressive renal insufficiency caused by obstruction, renal drainage (by stenting or nephrostomy) must be performed immediately.

Bladder TB stage 4 (microcystis) is indicated for cystectomy following by enteroplastic. Radical cystectomy with full removing fibrotic tissue is preferable, and after augmentation relapse and complication is more probable. Bladder and ureter reconstruction with ileum is a good option in difficult cases of lack or irreversible damage of the urinary way.

Keywords Urogenital tuberculosis • Surgery • Cystectomy • Enteroplastic • Endoscopic surgery

6.1 Introduction

UGTB like any other UTI may and should be cured conservatively (if it is diagnosed in-time). Surgical intervention is indicated for KTB 3–4 stages, for correction of complications (urinary tract tuberculosis). All surgical interventions should be performed on the background of anti-TB therapy, the exact time point will be estimated after histological investigation of the removed tissue (Kholtobin and Kulchavenya 2013; Singh et al. 2011; Suárez-Grau et al. 2012). In 17.9 % the caseous material was positive for acid-fast bacilli on direct smear (Wong and Lau 1980).

Neo-adjuvant anti-TB chemotherapy is strictly indicated for at least 2 months – in combination with pathogenetic therapy (Nguyen Phuc Cam Hoang et al. 2009;

E. Kulchavenya, *Current Therapy and Surgery for Urogenital Tuberculosis*,
DOI 10.1007/978-3-319-28290-9_6

Ngo Gia Hy 2000; Bennani et al. 1994). Positive experience of laparoendoscopic single-site nephrectomy using home-made single-port device for nonfunctioning kidney due to KTB was described (Han et al. 2010).

6.2 Indication for Surgery for UGTB Patients

6.2.1 Surgery for Kidney TB

Even in the era of modern anti-TB drugs, nephrectomy is still an essential procedure. It was recommended to perform early nephrectomy for patients with major renal lesion with or without bladder involvement, gross hydronephrosis and for those who have glomerular filtration rate (GFR) of <20 ml/min/m^2. Lower ureteral strictures and renal units with GFR of >20 ml/min/m^2 are favourable factors and salvage procedures are successful in these cases. It is likely that nephrectomy removes a large focus of disease and possibly dormant bacteria. With continuance of chemotherapy, this further helps in improved patient outcome (Viswaroop et al. 2006).

The surgical exploration should be done on all patients with non-functioning tuberculous kidneys to, (1) salvage kidneys before they are damaged totally by the obstructive lesions, (2) remove a potential source of infection with viable organisms and (3) shorten convalescence. Wong and Lau (1980) in 89.3 % of their UGTB patients have diagnosed complicated KTB 4th stage and performed them nephrectomy. In 10.7 % a reconstructive operation was possible with gratifying results (Wong and Lau 1980).

In a study of Fischer and Flamm (1990) of the 72 patients with urinary tuberculosis, 21 received exclusively conservative treatment, while 16 underwent conservative surgery and the remaining 35, ablational surgery. The high nephrectomy and overall operation rate was explained by the high percentage of advanced state of disease and a large number of patients referred to authors for nephrectomy following long-term conservative treatment. A retrospective justification for this procedure is found in the fact that 52 % of the surgical specimens showed florid tuberculosis, though the patients had been receiving standardized chemotherapy for an average of 9 months (Fischer and Flamm 1990).

Among 167 new-revealed UGTB patients 70 % were cured by chemotherapy, and surgery was indicated for the rest 30 %; as a whole 85.1 % recovered (Nguyen Phuc Cam Hoang et al. 1994). Other authors were not so optimistic. In their study 51 % of UGTB patients underwent surgery and in 73 % it was nephrectomy. Relatively in-time diagnostic allowed performing organ-saving operations to 9.4 % of patients only (Batyrov et al. 2004).

The organ-removing operations were performed in 73 % of UGTB patients (Batyrov et al. 2004). It was found that such eradicative techniques as nephrectomy and nephruretherectomy still prevail. Early drainage of the kidney for its decompression allows preservation of the kidney and following reconstructive surgery in 70.6 % of cases. The number of early and later complications considerably decreased (Zuban' et al. 2008).

6.2.2 Endoscopic Surgery for Kidney TB

Hemal et al. (2000) compared results of retroperitoneoscopic nephrectomy with open surgery for TB nonfunctioning kidneys. They performed retroperitoneoscopic nephrectomy for tuberculous nonfunctioning kidneys to nine patients, and to another nine patients – open nephrectomy. Retroperitoneoscopic nephrectomy was successful in seven of the nine patients. Although two of the patients required conversion to open surgery, the remaining seven successfully underwent retroperitoneoscopic nephrectomy after modifying the technique. The authors concluded that TB has been considered a contraindication to retroperitoneoscopic nephrectomy due to a high conversion rate. However, they believe that their modified technique of retroperitoneoscopic nephrectomy is a viable option for managing TB nonfunctioning kidneys (Hemal et al. 2000).

Lee et al. (2002) performed laparoscopic nephrectomy successfully on 30 patients with KTB as well as on 44 patients without TB (control group). The two groups showed comparable perioperative and postoperative parameters, except for mean operative time, which, at 244 min for the tuberculosis group, was significantly greater than the 216 min for the control group ($P<0.05$). No significant intraoperative or postoperative complications were observed in either group.

The results of this study indicate that laparoscopic nephrectomy for renal tuberculosis is a safe, effective, and less invasive treatment modality. Therefore Lee et al. (2002) suggested that the renal tuberculous nonfunctioning kidney should be approached initially using the laparoscopic approach.

Gupta et al. (1997) described a case of KTB 4th stage with a nonfunctioning kidney in which laparoscopic nephrectomy was attempted. The kidney was very difficult to mobilize due to dense perinephric adhesions (that is common for KTB 4th stage) and subsequently the procedure was converted to an open nephrectomy. The authors think KTB 4th stage is a relative contraindication to laparoscopic approach as its dissection is difficult and fraught with potential complications such as leakage of caseous material into the peritoneal cavity and systemic dissemination of the disease (Gupta et al. 1997).

Suárez-Grau et al. (2012) described their experience of laparoscopic surgery of an enterovesical fistula of tuberculous origin (terminal ileum and sigmoid colon).

6.2.3 Surgery for UGTB in Co-Morbidity with Urolithiasis

Due often to co-morbidity of KTB and stone disease, in a patient diagnosed with ureterolithiasis, a thorough history and physical examination, with specific attention to HIV and tuberculosis predisposing factors, should be carried out and preoperative screening tests considering the possibility of urinary tuberculosis are required. Finally, if urinary tuberculosis is detected, extracorporeal shock-wave lithotripsy must be postponed until after appropriate treatment of tuberculosis (Tourchi et al. 2014).

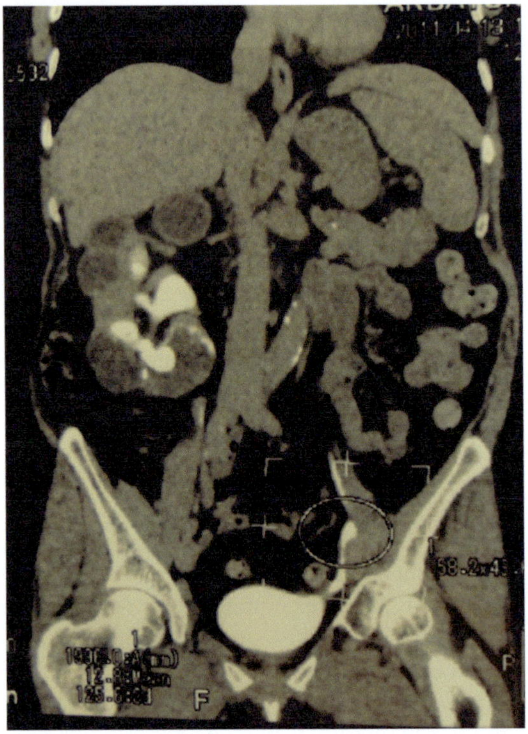

Fig. 6.1 Multi-slice computer tomogram – big stone in right kidney alongside with some huge caverns

I would like to present a case of co-morbidity of KTB 4th stage, bladder TB 4th stage as well as horny-like staghorn kidney stone. A female patient, 54 years of age, survived treatment and managed to be a typical patient with urolithiasis and chronic pyelonephritis for 10 years, and her urograms (Fig. 6.1) were interpreted as stone disease. Secondary to stone recurrent pyelonephritis was diagnosed with severe dysuria, pyuria, growth of Enterobacter spp10^7 CFU/ml in urine, first sensitive to all antibiotics. The patient was treated with fluoroquinolones and amicacin with a very short "cold" period with fast relapse of the disease. Lithotripsy was scheduled, but concerning IVU picture KTB was suspected, but bacteriology didn't reveal Mtb. It was not surprising, as she received in total 34 courses of antibiotics – mostly non-optimal antibiotics. Due to resistance to the therapy, the patient was admitted into the Urogenital Clinic of Novosibirsk Research TB Institute, and complex examination confirmed UGTB by clinic and laboratory tests; Mtb was found once by PCR.

The patient had bladder volume 40 ml with day frequency of urination 30–35, and nocturia 10–12 – but without incontinence.

The anti-TB chemotherapy was started, and in 2 months nephruretercystectomy on the right was performed with following enteroplastic (operation material is shown in Fig. 6.2). After surgery ChT was continued for 10 months with good efficiency. Follow up is 3 years, the patient retains wellbeing, dysuria and pyuria are absent, and function of urinary reservoir is satisfied.

It was the good fortune of our patient that extracorporeal shock-wave lithotripsy was not made before anti-TB ChT as haematogenous dissemination of undiagnosed urinary tuberculosis after performing extracorporeal shock-wave lithotripsy is high probable (Tourchi et al. 2014).

6.2.4 Surgery for Urinary Tract TB

Urinary tract TB is a complication of kidney TB which requires reconstructive surgery – if it is not done in time, results of the complex therapy are poor.

6.2.4.1 Surgery for Tuberculous Ureteral Stricture

Tuberculous ureteral stricture causing progressive obstructive uropathy commonly complicates KTB. Shin et al. (2002) reported on seventy-seven patients (84 renal units) with TB ureteral strictures. They evaluated the final outcome of involved kidneys with three different managements: medication only (n=37), medication plus ureteral stenting (n=28), or medication plus percutaneous nephrostomy (n=19). In spite of the complex therapy, the overall nephrectomy rate was high – 51 %. Expected biggest nephrectomy rate (73 %) was in patients treated with medication only, but in patients treated with medication plus early ureteral stenting or percutaneous nephrostomy the nephrectomy rate reduced twice – to 34 % (Shin et al. 2002).

The rate of reconstructive surgery for ureteral strictures also was significantly different for patients treated with medication only (8 %) and those receiving medication plus early ureteral stenting or percutaneous nephrostomy (49 %). Spontaneous resolution of the strictures was noted in six of the 12 renal units that were managed with early ureteral stenting. The authors concluded that early ureteral stenting or percutaneous nephrostomy in patients with TB ureteral strictures may increase the opportunity for later reconstructive surgery and decrease the likelihood of renal loss (Shin et al. 2002).

Current surgical techniques are highly effective in UGTB patients. Zuban' et al. (2014) performed surgical treatment on 92 patients with KTB, complicated by extended or multiple ureteral strictures. Thirty-five patients with nephrotuberculosis underwent percutaneous needle-guided nephrostomy, 79 underwent surgery with removal of organs: open nephrectomy with lumbar access (48), combined nephroureterectomy (31). According to the evaluation the glomerular filtration rate after nephrostomy, value less than 10 ml/min led to performing nephrectomy, more than 10 ml/min – ureteroplasty. It was established that combined nephroureterectomy has significant advantages in the case of specific kidney disease, despite a long duration as compared with a nephrectomy. Removal of the kidney with ureter in patient with nephrotuberculosis is the prevention of persistent dysuria, empyema of ureter stump, its possible malignant transformation, and contributes to significant improve-

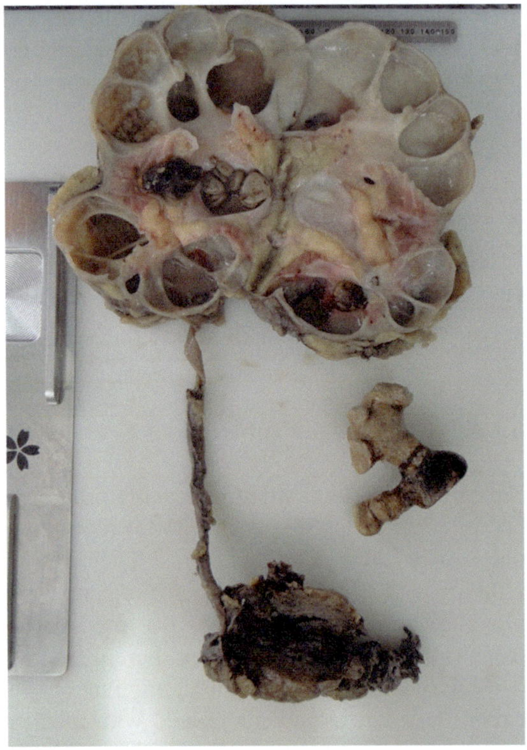

Fig. 6.2 Operation material of female patient, who suffered from KTB-4, bladder TB-4, stone disease, secondary chronic pyelonepfritis (Foto is prepared by Dr Denis Kholtobin)

ment of quality of life of the patient. Of the 35 patients after nephrostomy, 25 underwent intestinoplasty of ureter: ileum was used in 23 patients, appendix- in two patients. It is shown that reconstructive surgery using small intestine allows releasing 92 % of patients from a lifetime external drainage of the kidney.

Murav'ev and Zuban' (2012) presented the results of the surgery treatment of 73 patients with KTB complicated by ureteritis. Patients were divided into four groups. The first three groups underwent percutaneous puncture nephrostomy (1st group), open nephrostomy (2nd group) and internal stent placement (3rd group). Patients in group 4 were not operated. It was found that long-term ChT for UTTB patients leads to progressive urine retention resulted in loss of renal function in 63 % of cases. Early urine diversion, depending on its method, allows preserving the functional ability of the kidneys in 70.8 to 94.4 % of cases. The combination of early renal drainage with anti-TB chemotherapy is significantly superior to conservative treatment only. At the same time, good results of plastics were achieved only in patients undergoing a two-stage surgical treatment, and poor results (relapse of stricture, progression of hydroureteronephrosis or CRF) were significantly more often observed (60 %) in patients without urine diversion (Murav'ev and Zuban' 2012).

To assess the effect of the relief of obstruction on the ultimate function of the affected renal unit in urinary tuberculosis, and to identify predictors of functional recoverability, Ramanathan et al. (1998) of a total of 38 patients with urinary tuberculosis with evidence of upper tract obstruction have analyzed. Six patients had bilateral obstruction (total of 44 renal units). Ten renal units were not functioning, and no preliminary intervention was performed. In the remaining 34, preliminary intervention was carried out before definitive surgery; 21 of these renal units were salvaged but 13 were lost despite overcoming the obstruction. The authors have found that the loss of some renal units seems inevitable in UGTB patients, despite advances in chemotherapy. Having pre-operative predictors of renal recovery may ensure optimal patient selection, thereby reducing the number of procedures and economic burden on the patient who does not require intervention (Ramanathan et al. 1998).

6.2.4.2 Surgery for Bladder TB

One of the reasons of low efficacy of anti-TB therapy for complicated KTB is overfibrosis resulting in development of ureteral stricture and bladder contraction. Bladder TB in terminal stage (microcystis or thimble bladder) may be fatal disease. Development of contracted bladder is indication for operation, but there is no unique approach to surgery.

Bladder TB stage 4 (microcystis) is indicated for cystectomy following by enteroplastic (Kholtobin and Kulchavenya 2013). Urinary bladder rehabilitation either by augmentation cystoplasty or orthotopic neobladder reconstruction increases the bladder capacity and storage time and also preserves the upper tracts (Singh et al. 2011). I'd like to note, that radical cystectomy with full removing fibrotic tissue is preferable, and after augmentation relapse and complication are more probable. Bladder and ureter reconstruction with ileum is a good option in difficult cases of lack or irreversible damage of the urinary way. Vesico-ureteral reconstruction letting urethral miction improves quality of life (Resina et al. 2009). Patients after full course of the therapy and, if it was indicated, surgery, should be under surveillance for 3–5 years with annual check-up and anti-relapse therapy, if necessary.

Twenty nine patients with contracted TB bladder (4th stage) were admitted in the urogenital clinic of Novosibirsk Research TB Institute for reconstructive surgery; 27 patients had natural bladder TB and two patients had BCG-inducted contracted bladder. Male patients were 10 (34.5 %); female patients were 19 (65.5 %). The median age was 55.6 (range 28–70 years old). Nephrectomy for kidney TB was performed on 6 (20.7 %) patients earlier. Female patients underwent partial cystectomy (subtrigonal – 18 patients, supratrigonal –1 patient). The spectrum of operations in male patients was as followed: cystprostatectomy in six patients, prostate-sparing cystectomy in one patient, augmentation ileocystoplasty in one patient and radical cystectomy in two patients with BCG-induced bladder TB. Orthotopic neobladder was reconstructed by the Studer method.

Results of the surgery were estimated as good (bladder volume 400 ml and more without frequency, incontinence and residual urine), moderate (bladder volume

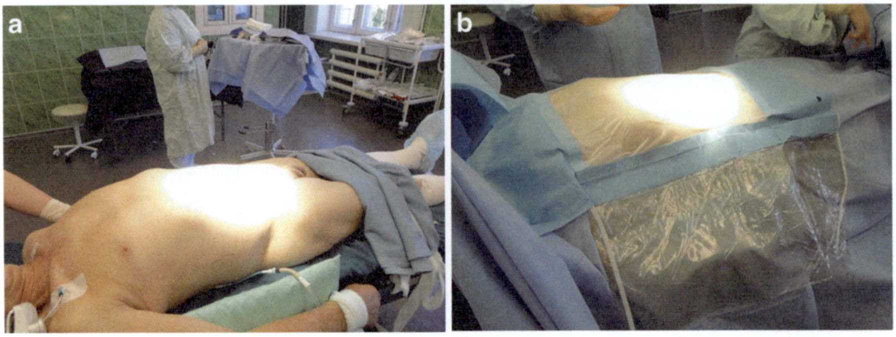

Fig. 6.3 Approach for cystectomy: (**a**) – position of the patient on a surgical table; (**b**) – skin is covered by sterile tissue (Fotos are prepared by Dr Denis Kholtobin)

400 ml, but there is recurrent urinary infection, residual urine requiring intermitted catheterization, late surgical complications), and poor (insufficient bladder volume, progressive renal failure).

A good result was achieved in 22 patients (76 %), moderate in six (21 %) and one (3 %) patient had poor result. Among six patients with moderate result one male patient after augmentation ileocystoplasty had irritation and residual urine. To solve these complications he was re-operated in 11 months: cystprostatectomy with Studer neobladder was performed. Follow up showed good result. Although one female patient had no good result as she had frequent urination (10–13 per day), nocturia was 2–3 times per night – but she was satisfied because before surgical treatment she urinated 45–55 times daily. Two female patients had stricture of ureteral-neovesical anastomosis and recurrent infection and anastomosis was re-done in a 6 month period. Two female patients had evacuatory disorders resulting in residual urine and symptomatic recurrent infection. One of them had pelvic organ prolapse and underwent open mesh-sacrovaginopexy that improved her condition. Self-catheterization was recommended to another one, where there was no anatomical reason for surgery. One male patient after prostate-sparing cystectomy had poor results: progressive renal failure, evacuatory disorders, residual urine. He had comorbidity HIV-infection and we suppose it may be a reason for a poor result (Kholtobin et al. 2014). Stages of the cystectomy and result of the operation in one of our patient is shown below (Figs. 6.3, 6.4, 6.5, 6.6, 6.7, 6.8, and 6.9).

Dogra et al. (2014) performed the technique of robot-assisted laparoscopic augmentation ileocystoplasty in a patient with a small contracted bladder due to UGTB via a completely intra-corporeal technique using an ileal "cap" created from a 15 cm segment of distal ileum which was anastomosed to the urinary bladder bi-valved in the mid-sagittal plane. The procedure lasted for 420 min and the patient was discharged on postoperative day 5. Although in 6 months the patient had no irritative urinary symptoms and urinated with insignificant post-void

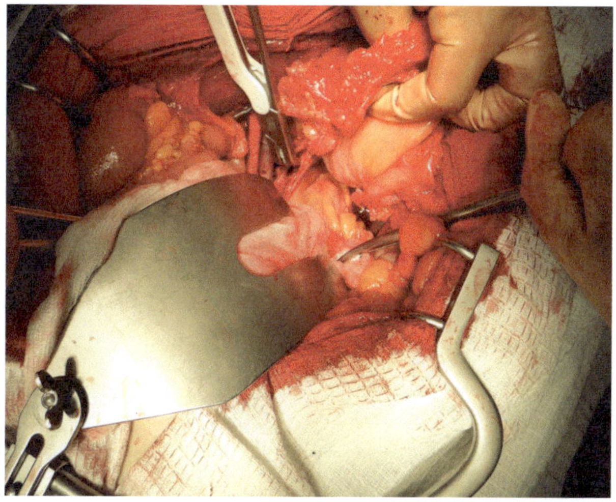

Fig. 6.4 A stage of an operation – a processing of lateral bladder wall by Ligasure (Foto is prepared by Dr Denis Kholtobin)

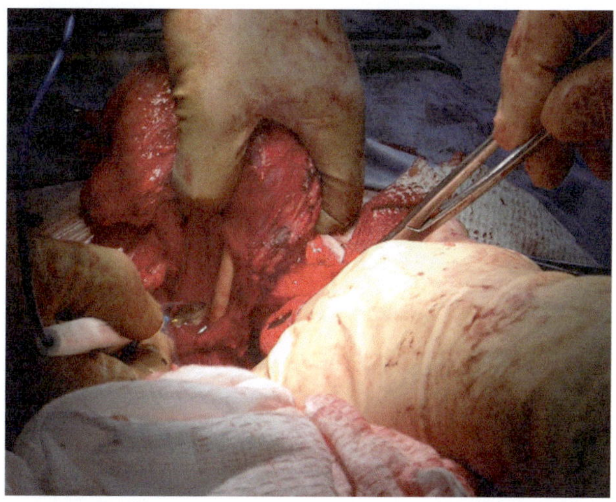

Fig. 6.5 Subtrigonal cystectomy (Foto is prepared by Dr Denis Kholtobin)

residual urine, we cannot be sure of a lasting good effect. Augmentation ileocystoplasty is not an optimal operation for UGTB patients as full, radical removing of fibrous tissue is indicated, and otherwise a likelihood of complication and relapse is high.

Cutaneous fistula revealing tubercular pyonephrosis was described (Elkihal et al. 2010), and possibility of retroperitoneoscopic nephrectomy for tuberculous nephrocolonic fistula. This operation was found to be feasible and safe (Modi and Rizvi 2008).

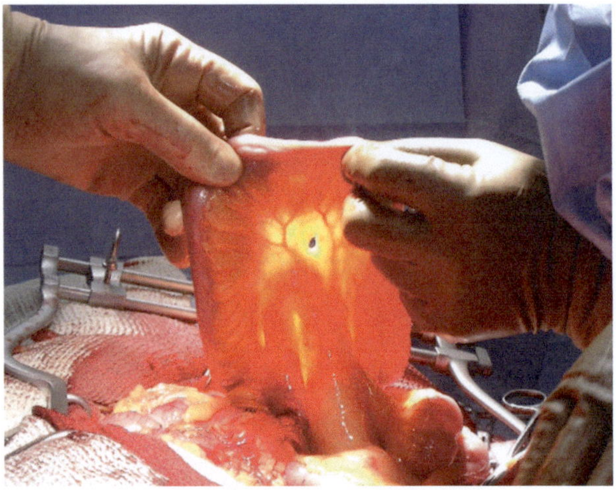

Fig. 6.6 Releasing of ileum segment (Foto is prepared by Dr Denis Kholtobin)

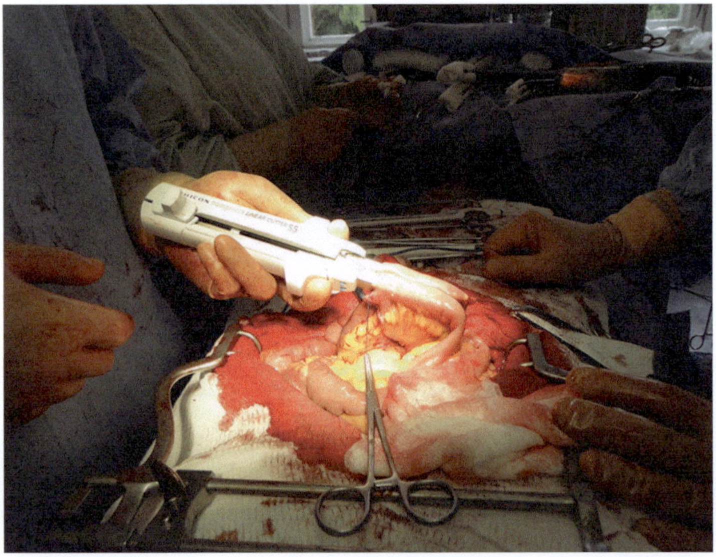

Fig. 6.7 Isoperistaltic side-to-side anastomosis (Foto is prepared by Dr Denis Kholtobin)

Summary of recommendation on surgical intervention for UGTB patients is shown in Table 6.1.

6.3 Conclusion

Despite really great success of chemotherapy for UGTB, there is a number of patients who have to be treated by surgery. The reasons for the limit on the medications are:

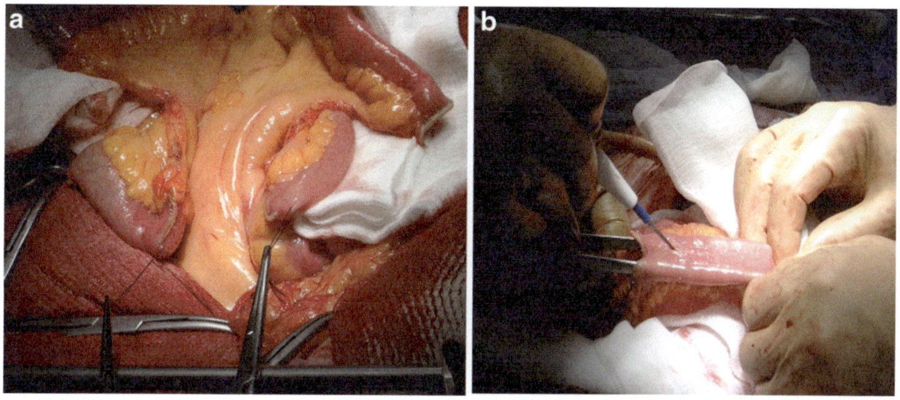

Fig. 6.8 Stages of a detubularisation of ileum: (**a**) – the ileum is fixed, (**b**) – a detubularisation with electrosurgical instrument (Fotos are prepared by Dr Denis Kholtobin)

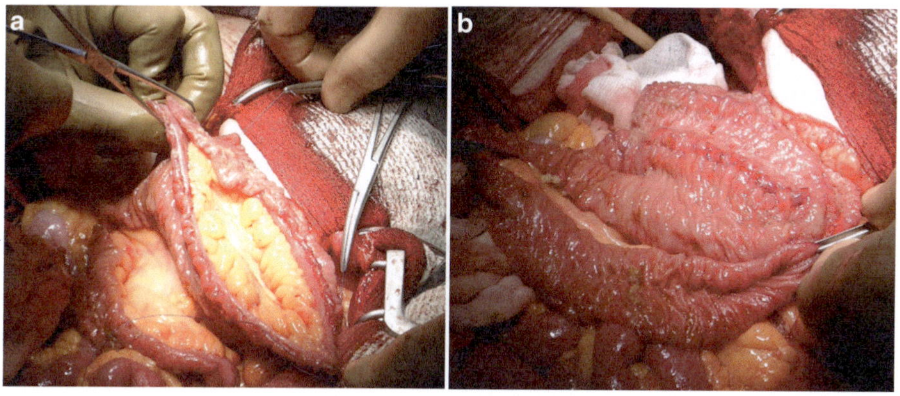

Fig. 6.9 Formation of reservoir: (**a**) – first stage and (**b**) –final stage (Fotos are prepared by Dr Denis Kholtobin)

1. Late diagnosis. If the patient is revealed in first stages – he will be cured by ant-YB drugs, but if he is revealed late, with complication – surgery is inevitable.
2. Non-optimal chemotherapy. Using streptomycin in sub-optimal doses, neglecting the pathogenetic therapy may lead to development overfibrosis and disorder or even loss of the function of the organ.

Possibilities of current surgical techniques may help any patient, nevertheless the best operation is an operation which has been avoided.

Table 6.1 Surgical treatment for UGTB

Indication	Surgery
1. Kidney TB:	
KTB-3, resistant to standard therapy (notably cavern with pyogenic layer remains, Mtb in urine, pyuria) for 2–4 months	Cavernectomy (partial nephrectomy), optimal – laparoscopically.
KTB-4	Nephrectomy, optimal – laparoscopically
2. Urinary tract tuberculosis:	
Stricture of ureter, urethra	Standard plastic operation
Bladder TB 4 stage	Cystectomy (in male patients – cystprostatectomy) with following enteroplastic by standard technique.
3. TB orchiepididymitis:	
Fluctuation, abscess	Incision of abscess and drainage
Torpid course with low efficiency of conservative treatment for 1–2 months	Orchidectomy
4. Prostate TB (normally prostate TB is not indicated for surgery):	
Development of abscess	Drainage of abscess

References

Batyrov FA, Nersesian AA, Merkur'eva IA (2004) Urogenital tuberculosis: problems of present-day diagnosis and treatment. Urologiia 5:16–24

Bennani S, Aboutaieb R, el Mrini M, Benjelloun S (1994) The role of corticotherapy and endoscopy in the treatment of urogenital tuberculosis. Ann Urol (Paris) 28(5):243–249

Dogra PN, Regmi SK, Singh P, Bora G, Saini AK, Aggarwal S (2014) Robot-assisted laparoscopic augmentation ileocystoplasty in a tubercular bladder. Urol Ann 6(2):152–155. doi:10.4103/0974-7796.130647

Elkihal N, Senouci K, Hassam B, Ismaili N (2010) Cutaneous fistula revealing tubercular pyonephrosis. Ann Dermatol Venereol 137(8–9):580–581

Fischer M, Flamm J (1990) The value of surgical therapy in the treatment of urogenital tuberculosis. Urologe 29(5):261–264

Gupta NP, Agrawal AK, Sood S (1997) Tubercular pyelonephritic nonfunctioning kidney–another relative contraindication for laparoscopic nephrectomy: a case report. J Laparoendosc Adv Surg Tech A 7(2):131–134

Han WK, Park YH, Jeon HG (2010) The feasibility of laparoendoscopic single-site nephrectomy: initial experience using home-made single-port device. Urology 76(4):862–865

Hemal AK, Gupta NP, Rajeev TP, Kumar R, Dar L, Seth P (2000) Polymerase chain reaction in clinically suspected genitourinary tuberculosis: comparison with intravenous urography, bladder biopsy, and urine acid fast bacilli culture. Urology 56(4):570–574

Kholtobin D, Kulchavenya EV (2013) Surgery for bladder tuberculosis. Palmarium Academium Publishing, Berlin, 76 p

Kholtobin DP, Kulchavenya EV, Khomyakov VT (2014) Bladder TB 4-th stage – how to improve urination? Urologia 5:26–29

Lee KS, Kim HH, Byun SS, Kwak C, Park K, Ahn H (2002) Laparoscopic nephrectomy for tuberculous nonfunctioning kidney: comparison with laparoscopic simple nephrectomy for other diseases. Urology 60(3):411–414

Modi PR, Rizvi SJ (2008) Retroperitoneoscopic nephrectomy for nephrocolonic fistula due to tuberculous nonfunctioning kidney. J Laparoendosc Adv Surg Tech A 18(6):841–843

Murav'ev AN, Zuban' ON (2012) Role of supravesicular urine diversion in the treatment of patients with renal and urethraltuberculosis. Urologiia 6:16–20

Ngo Gia Hy (2000) Overview on genitourinary tuberculosis. Ho Chi Minh city's Medico-pharmacology Actualities. pp 68–72

Nguyen Phuc Cam Hoang, Cam Hoang, Pham Van Bui, Vo Thi Hong Lien (1994) A propos of 167 cases of genitourinary tuberculosis treated at Binh Dan hospital in 5 years. Binh Dan Hospital's Sci Technol Actualities 7:293–305

Nguyen Phuc Cam Hoang, Le Van Hieu Nhan, Phan Van Hoang, Tran Ngoc Khac Linh, & Vu Le Chuyen (2009) Are tuberculosis nonfunctioning kidneys amenable to laparoscopic nephrectomy? (Abstract), Urology 74 (Supplement 4A), 30th Congress of the Société Internationale d'Urologie, S189

Ramanathan R, Kumar A, Kapoor R, Bhandari M (1998) Relief of urinary tract obstruction in tuberculosis to improve renal function. Analysis of predictive factors. Br J Urol 81(2):199–205

Resina RG, Ruiz BC, López RA, Romero FJ (2009) Complete vesico-ureteral reconstruction with ileum in a case of genitourinary Tuberculosis. Actas Urol Esp 33(6):706–711

Shin KY, Park HJ, Lee JJ, Park HY, Woo YN, Lee TY (2002) Role of early endourologic management of tuberculous ureteral strictures. J Endourol 16(10):755–758

Singh V, Sinha RJ, Sankhwar SN, Sinha SM (2011) Reconstructive surgery for tuberculous contracted bladder: experience of a center in northern India. Int Urol Nephrol 43(2):423–430

Suárez-Grau JM, Bellido-Luque JA, Pastrana-Mejía A, Gómez-Menchero J, García-Moreno JL, Durán-Ferreras I (2012) Guadalajara-Jurado JF Laparoscopic surgery of an enterovesical fistula of tuberculous origin (terminal ileum and sigmoid colon). Rev Esp Enferm Dig 104(7):391–392

Tourchi A, Ebadi M, Hosseinzadeh A, Shabaninia M (2014) Disseminated tuberculosis after extracorporeal shock-wave lithotripsy in an AIDS patient presenting with urosepsis. Int J STD AIDS 25(3):231–234. doi:10.1177/0956462413498580. Epub 2013 Aug 1

Viswaroop B, Gopalakrishnan G, Nath V, Kekre NS (2006) Role of imaging in predicting salvageability of kidneys in urinary tract tuberculosis. J Pak Med Assoc 56(12):587–590

Wong SH, Lau WY (1980) The surgical management of non-functioning tuberculous kidneys. J Urol 124(2):187–191

Zuban' ON, Murav'ev AN, Volkov AA, (2008) Surgical treatment of nephrotuberculosis in the present-day epidemiological situation. Vestn Khir Im I I Grek 167(1):92–95

Zuban' ON, Skorniakov SN, Arkanov LV, Novikov BI, Chotchaev RM (2014) Surgical treatment of tuberculosis of the kidney with a total lesion of the ureter. Urologiia 2:29–33

MIX
Papier aus verantwortungsvollen Quellen
Paper from responsible sources
FSC® C105338

If you have any concerns about our products,
you can contact us on
ProductSafety@springernature.com

In case Publisher is established outside the EU,
the EU authorized representative is:
Springer Nature Customer Service Center GmbH
Europaplatz 3, 69115 Heidelberg, Germany

Printed by Libri Plureos GmbH
in Hamburg, Germany